D0796510

DON'T WAIT UNTIL YOU'RE SICK

How Research-Based Healing can Double as Prevention

AARON GROSSKOPF

ISBN- 978-0578403649

Printed in the United States of America

LIFEINSURANCEBUYERS.COM

I f the unfortunate does come upon you or a loved one and you find yourself in the fight of your life, it can take a quick toll, mentally, physically, and spiritually. These stresses don't make things any easier. Throw on top of that hefty medical bills and the burden can become more immense. Life Insurance buyers can buy your policy and supply you with a percentage of what it is worth to aid in medical bills when fighting a disease.

I have no affiliation with them, but this info could be a tremendous help to anyone fighting for their lives. This is a prime example for the basis of this book, spreading knowledge that most people would otherwise never hear or think about.

Peace

DEDICATION

There are many that have gone before us. Dad (Jim Grosskopf) and Kevin Rowland, I wish I knew then what I know now. Cheers some Chard, and point this to those who are ready and need it.

Thank you to those who are mentioned in this book, and those who aren't. It's a brave, just cause to dedicate yourself to helping others heal, which can also be met with fierce opposition.

Back cover photo credit to Katie Newburn @cloudsandcoffee
Cover design by Anthony Kimball @ authorcreative.com

CONTENTS

INTRODUCTION

Something Is Ass-Backwards in America Today

I know, what an introduction, but seriously, our great nation is the sickest it has ever been. In the last 30-50 years, heart disease and cancer have become the top two causes of death we face today. What happened? Yes, those diseases were around 50 years ago, but things should have improved by now. Why haven't they?

One broad answer, and this is by no means a general assumption, is that a majority of our health care professionals have not been adequately trained in prevention and/or nutrition.[1]

My Epiphany

In 2006, my uncle (my dad's brother; they're together again) was struck by lung cancer. He went through the conventional treatments. It may have been too late, the treatments may not have worked, I'm not sure. But during his suffering, all that I remember thinking is, "There must be something else that can be done to help. In the whole wide world, there is nothing that can be done? That doesn't sit right."

I stumbled upon a story of a husband and wife. The husband had cancer – can't remember what kind, what stage, or if they were 100% holistic, but it was bad.

The epiphany was his wife would juice broccoli for him several times a day. Broccoli! He got better and went into remission. I'm sure that there were other factors, and I'm not saying broccoli juice cures cancer, or that there is any silver bullet, but I definitely woke up to the fact that there are other ways to treat disease and, as in most cases, some of these holistic treatments are preventative as well.

> *"Horse, meet water."*
> *- Porter Stansberry*

I want to give you some LOVE

This is the point of this book. Many holistic therapies, treatments, remedies, and protocols can be used to fight disease in the body. They can also be great preventatives that are non-toxic with minimal to no side effects and can help you live a long healthy life. I'm going to touch on these in this book and hopefully inspire you to open some rabbit holes of your own. I want to open your eyes to true healing and how the body intends it to happen.

> *"When you truly heal, the whole body heals"*
> *-Charlotte Gerson[2]*

Imagine that you're at the doctor's office, and a test comes back saying that you have high cholesterol. The doctor will most likely prescribe a class of prescriptions called Statin, which comes with a list of possible side effects, including cancer.[3]

Most likely, anyone with a preventative, holistic mindset would instead adopt a plant-based diet. This includes replacing the LDL-causing fats like canola, corn, and vegetable oils with HDL-promoting oils like avocado, coconut, and olive oil. Furthermore, the use of lavender, lemongrass, and rosemary essential oils, internally and externally, is helpful in balancing out cholesterol levels. And that's just to start!

I want to give you some more LOVE

Statin might be the easiest, most readily available, well-known option that is covered by insurance – and may be a part of the bigger problem. These statins work on the symptoms, but they do not address the root cause of the problem. I want to show you examples of how the second option of treatment, which may take some extra effort, has the possibility to prevent other conditions as well. Would you be willing to do some extra work if you knew you could address one issue while preventing others from happening?

June 8, 2018 – I woke up this morning, popped open my phone to see what was going on in the world, and the first picture I see is of Anthony Bourdain with the text "RIP". What a shock; being a chef myself and seeing the outpouring of grief from the culinary world, it's a big hit. The holistic side of me couldn't help but think what pharmaceuticals were in his travel bag. If this was indeed a suicide. Point being, there are non-pharmaceutical, holistic approaches that can balance hormones and treat anxiety and depression.

One simple example is curcumin, which is found in the spice turmeric.[4,5,6] Curcumin is also an anti-inflammatory, which can ease inflamed arteries and aid in the prevention of cardiovascular issues.[7]

Show me the money! Or the LOVE

I have the utmost respect and compassion for any person or any family who has lost a loved one or is in the fight of their lives with cancer. I also feel it is a grand gesture to honor them by supporting a cause. At the same time, there is a big message that is not reaching the majority.

This introduction was first drafted on June 7, 2018. Earlier in the day when I was putting some bullet points together, I found myself on the official Pink Ribbon website. For years, I was a private chef in San Diego, California. I would shop at Whole Foods and drive to the boss's house to cook. There was always a time of year where I would be stopped at an intersection in La Jolla. I was in a hurry to get dinner started, but the parade of the pink walk wouldn't stop coming, God bless them! It would be almost eight minutes before traffic control would make a break for cars.

That's where the question arose - where does all the money go that is raised toward cancer research? I thought it would be easy to find. I thought it would be in bright pink on the home page: "Your dollars funded this study" or "Your dollars are funding this research". It's not there; I couldn't find anything but a generic statement in the FAQ.

Why am I picking on Pink?
Don't worry, I'm going to pick on Avon too

My intent here isn't to strike a negative tone. My hope is to spread knowledge and make the introduction so that YOU truly have the power to heal and to find what works for you to take your health into your own hands.

Ladies, please, please, please be aware of what you are lathering all over your face and body!

If one person goes into their vanity kit and takes a good look at the ingredients on their makeup or lotion, that is a good starting point to prevention.[8]

Here is where I, and hopefully you, take issue with the products that are made for Pink, which is raising awareness for cancer. I read an article about a mother and daughter who were wondering the same thing as they were scooping ice cream with a pink scooper: where does the money go? Why on earth would you associate ice cream with cancer awareness? Sugar is the main fuel source and driver of cancer growth.[9] I felt sorry for them. Had no one told them this fact? Their doctor, their oncologist? This is double wrong.

Pink Avon Lipstick … Selling pink lipstick where some of the proceeds go to cancer research? Awareness? Detection? Protection? The cosmetic industry uses all sorts of carcinogenic (cancer-causing) ingredients in their products. Where do these toxins end up after being applied and absorbed? What kind of issues can they cause? The irony of selling a toxic product and slapping a pink ribbon on it should infuriate people.[10, 11]

Per my epiphany, I started to dig, I've researched holistic therapies and approaches far and wide, and I would tell myself, "Well, if it ever comes, I feel equipped to take action." I'm a chef, and in my recent past, I didn't have the best diet. I liked to party more than I should have, I didn't drink a lot of water, had some stress, and didn't really exercise. I was overweight as well, but nothing life-threatening.

I moved from San Diego back home to the Bay Area in San Francisco, along with my girlfriend at the time, still chugging along, still researching and remaining interested in alternative therapies, living an almost healthy lifestyle. We broke up, and a few months later, she was diagnosed with stage IV breast cancer. I knew what to do, but she decided on another route. She is in remission and doing well as far as I know; I wish her and her family the best.

This was a huge wake-up call. If someone that I had spent almost every day with and lived an almost identical lifestyle with got this sick, where does that leave me? As synchronicity would have it, I had discovered The Truth about Cancer and their movement, all with in the Months this was playing out. I went to their first live event, and I watched Dr. David Jockers speak, and this is where a big change happened in my life. I dropped almost 30 pounds, felt great, and switched my metabolism over to burn clean energy, naturally, using nutrition. I'm not a doctor or a nutritionist; I don't have a

PhD, but on my own I learned and found a path to feeling the best I have probably ever felt, and you can do it too.

This sparked some passion, and I became a Certified Holistic Integrative Health Coach through the Institute for Integrative Nutrition (IIN) out of New York City. Joshua Rosenthal's school was another life changer. Here, I learned balance and all the other principles of IIN. I highly recommend that you take the Health Coach Training program. It's worth it just to get yourself right!

These last two paragraphs are great examples of how the following writing will be laid out. I'll show you nontoxic, minimal-to-no side effects, natural treatments, remedies, and protocols that can fight and prevent disease, all at the same time. I want to get you to a point of Charlotte Gerson's whole-body healing.

There will be science, name-dropping, and citations for you to do research and come up with your own conclusion, but I will tell you one thing: you will end this book with a greater outlook of what you yourself can do to feel the best you have felt.

Of course, if you need a nudge, some accountability, or coaching, I'm here for ya. Bigheadhealth@gmail.com. My last name is Grosskopf.

It's German - it means Bighead ☺

've been in the room during the first consultation fresh after a cancer diagnosis. I don't have to tell you, but this is not a place that you want to be. For around two hours, you sit through a barrage of visits from case managers, social workers, and 3-4 different doctors, each with their own take on how they cut, burn, and poison you. In this case, the surgeon's and radiologist's work would come down the road, but the oncologist needs to start the chemo as soon as possible.

It seemed that there was no question that anyone could ask that could bring up other possible therapy options. There is no time to research, no time for second opinions; it's chemo now.

Most cancerous tumors are not something that grow overnight. It may take years for the cells to multiply into a size where they could be given a stage classification.[1] It's important to know that, even if you have a fast-growing tumor. In most cases, you have time to research your options and resist the pressure to start chemo, surgery, or radiation immediately.

Hopefully, what's discussed in the following pages can encourage you to look at other options when it comes to a cancer diagnosis. God forbid that day ever comes, but if it does for you or a loved one, wouldn't you want to be equipped with the knowledge of alternative treatments? Wouldn't you want knowledge you could share with a loved one? Wouldn't you want the chance to make an informed decision and not be rushed into toxic treatments that have the potential to kill you faster than the disease?[2,3] (Citation 2 is an old article, but its thesis still stands.)

Or, if you do decide to go forward with conventional treatments, wouldn't you want to be knowledgeable in ways to support yourself and your immune system through these therapies? If conventional treatments are successful and an oncologist tells you, "We got it all," take it with a grain of salt. You may have had the tumors treated, and hopefully you've addressed the issue that made the tumors grow, but in most cases, the root cause is not addressed. Or, if the gauntlet of conventional treatments is unsuccessful, or a relapse occurs and you hear the words, "There is nothing more we can do," wouldn't you want to know that there absolutely are treatments that you can do?

Moreover, wouldn't you want to be equipped with the knowledge of how to lead a life where you give cancerous cells a slim chance of development or survival in the first place?

EMOTIONAL STRESS

In the beginning of researching alternative cancer treatments, I came across the Indie filmmaker Ian Jacklyn. A former kickboxing champion, actor, cancer coach, and a unique individual, Ian once had a girlfriend, Cynthia, who cured herself of cancer naturally. He made a documentary with her and others showing that they had cured themselves. They titled the documentary *icurecancer.com*. (Yes, that's the title.)

Cynthia Brooks rejected conventional (chemo, surgery, radiation) treatments. One of her key focuses was on spiritual and mental work, which is a big part of the cancer fight, holistic or conventional. Reducing stress, finding forgiveness, letting go, and getting out of that dead-end toxic relationship are all ways to help the body heal, to fight and prevent. This is where you can truly find root causes of what ails you. Stresses of these types can suppress the immune system, rendering the body vulnerable to imbalance and disease.

Everyone is different, everyone has different issues. So, talking it through is the one obvious way to address an imbalance. Speaking to therapists, psychiatrists, and even coaches or health coaches will help. As Joshua Rosenthal would tell us during our health coach training (and this is not a direct quote), "It takes someone who knows how to ask the right questions to create that Aha! moment."

I sometimes address acute stress easily by breathing. If someone makes you angry or you are behind and late for a project, you can feel the immediate stress. That feeling is a fight or flight response that triggers your immune system, and in turn can cause inflammation (we will cover this more later). I'll admit to getting stressed in the car; it used to take nothing to set me off, but I'm actively working on it. When a bout of anger or rage is triggered in a person, the sympathetic nervous system is activated; it's the fight or flight response, and a major stress. If this acute stress happens regularly, it can turn into chronic stress and chronic inflammation.

The flip side to this is the parasympathetic nervous system. It's the resting nervous system that is activated when you are in a calmer state. This nervous system is usually triggered when you're eating, digesting, at rest, or sexually aroused. It's an energy-conservation state of being.

When you feel stress and a fight or flight response kicks in, you can activate your parasympathetic nervous system on the spot by breathing. Realize the stress, identify it, feel it, then concentrate on your breathing. You are probably having short elevated breaths. Feel them and slow them down by taking big deep breaths. Feel your stomach expand when you breathe in deep, and feel it contract as you exhale. Breathe in through the nose and out through the mouth and focus on it. In about five seconds, you will have addressed that stress and kicked on your parasympathetic nervous system!

Addressing emotional stress is a key factor in balancing life and fighting disease. This emotional stress can run very deep: anything from the recent loss of a loved one to a received form of abuse that can stem back years or decades. It also could be stress you experience daily, like in a job or an abusive relationship.

I'm hesitant to write about the following. It's something I only share with close friends or loved ones. But it is an everyday example of this topic which I believe that you will benefit from.

My father passed in September 2017, and as of this writing, I still can't believe he is gone. I know the effects of death, and I knew that I had to take care of myself spiritually and mentally; it's something that I'm also actively working on. You never really get over a loss like that as many know, and it can take years to work through. This was obviously stress for my mom, sister, and myself. But my mom had another type of stress to deal with as well.

My parents were married very shortly after they met. They didn't know each other very well. I'll keep it brief: they should have been separated decades ago. They stayed together for us kids, I imagine. There was stress every day in my mother's life, maybe for my dad, too; they were in a toxic relationship.

My mother suffered from a lot of health ailments, and I was working with her to better her health toward the end of my dad's life. She really couldn't leave the house, had a very limited diet that she could handle, and was on a lot of prescription meds. Ever since my dad's passing, my mom has basically followed a plant-based ketogenic diet and used hemp to wean herself off doctor-prescribed narcotics. We go out to dinner; she finds herself dancing and singing at home with her puppies; we have a beer on the porch in the back yard. Mom was addressing health issues with diet and holistic measures to get off prescription drugs. But things, as sad as it is to say, got even better after dad died. The biggest stress in her life was gone.

These examples are all what suppress the immune system and host a toxic, acidic environment in the body. There are a couple of experts that I associate with in mental and spiritual healing, specifically when it comes to fighting cancer or other diseases.

The first is Dr. Veronique Desaulniers. She is known as the "Breast Cancer Conqueror" and has "seven steps" to healing breast cancer naturally. One of the steps involves emotional work and balance, which are just as important as everything else when addressing disease.

The second is Dr. Darrell Wolfe. He is known as the "Doc of Detox", and is a funny, passionate doctor who addresses toxicity on a mental and physical level. I believe his favorite word is Love, "vitamin L", and is a big proponent of "loving yourself."

Another expert that has loads of knowledge when it comes to the cancer fight is Chris Wark. The first time I encountered Chris was at a speaking engagement in Dallas, Texas at the Truth About Cancer Ultimate Live Symposium. Chris is a funny, lively young speaker who, after surgery on his stage III colon cancer, denied all other conventional treatments and healed himself naturally with nutrition and lots of mental work.

Chris's story really stuck in my head because he used techniques toward whole body healing at a time when the internet was new and everything that you are reading here was not readily available at your fingertips. After making his decision to fight naturally, Chris realized that everyone he knew who had supported him was against his decision to go holistic or natural. He is an exceptional story and a very strong individual to essentially go it alone.

The main reason I use Chris's story is to share his cancer coaching and general coaching programs. I listened to his multi-part series and have the materials he gives as a part of his program. There is nowhere else you would want to go for information directly after a cancer diagnosis than his program Square One.

He provides support, which is crucial, and even goes as far as giving a "20 questions for your oncologist" list. As I mentioned above, the initial appointments fresh after a cancer diagnosis are not something you want to go through. Unless you are pre-prepped for this, you will be unprepared for these meetings. Chemo, radiation, and surgery are presented in a way that puts a lot of pressure on you to make rash, life-altering decisions before you have a chance to start processing the diagnosis. Yes, there may be cases or emergency situations where you have no time. But most cancers take a long time to develop and they won't kill you overnight. Take the time to research and think about what is best for you, and remember Square One.

Specific examples of treatments to fight or prevent disease are just one way to aid yourself because there is no single cure. It's the combination that can assist in whole body healing, the only true cure. There are many who would look at that statement and roll their eyes at the quackery, or any mention of holistic treatments. That's fine, and I'm not here to debate. To each their own. I've learned from natural doctors, researchers, PhD's, professors, and the stories of the people they have helped, as well as contributing science.

ALKALINE DIET

an Jacklyn's mentor, Dr. Bernardo Majalca, has been called a quack, ridiculed in the mainstream media, and even jailed for treating patients with success in the U.S. when he wasn't allowed to. His treatment focused on getting the body back to an alkaline pH.

Dr. Bernardo's theory was that cancer patients were dying of acidosis, which can happen when the body reaches a pH of 5 - 5.5, which is an acidic state.[4] His alkaline diet would get the pH back up to a 7 - 7.5 alkalinity. Most of his cases were the worst out there. People usually found Dr. Bernardo after they had been diagnosed and gone through the gauntlet of conventional treatments, and either the cancer had come back or the patient didn't respond to treatments.

The doctors had basically sent the patients home to die because they felt that there was nothing more they could do.

After going through such harsh toxic treatments, it's no wonder the patients were so acidic; they had been poisoned! Dr. Bernardo's immediate first move is to get the patient drinking lemon water. Lemon and lime juice are acids, and there are arguments as to whether they can aid in alkalinity when they enter the body. Dr. Bernardo's protocol was juicing and forms of supplementation, an alkaline diet if you will. The argument is whether an alkaline diet has health benefits[5], but this kind of diet requires the consumption of mostly fruits and vegetables, along with their juices. I don't think we need a scientific journal to review the benefits of this.[6] For some, this diet was their saving grace to help the body heal and replenish lacking nutrients, and for most of us, it should be on the top of our list to prevent diseases.

need to give credit where credit is due and hopefully show people an eye-opening organization that could absolutely change or save your life or that of a friend or loved one. The organization is The Truth About Cancer. Ty and Charlene Bollinger created this movement as a book, then a docuseries, and now they even have a conference where all the doctors, scientists, professors, and experts who contributed to the series come to speak and also meet with the audience. These are the true rock stars of the natural health world, and they've had a profound impact on my life.

After losing his father, mother, and other family members to cancer, Ty realized that it was the treatments that had taken the lives of his loved ones. Not to say that cancer wouldn't have eventually taken their lives, but the treatments definitely sped up the process, or possibly did the damage themselves. This sparked his research and thus created the movement.

The amount of information that I have learned through this organization truly changed my life. I've sat next to cancer fighters, survivors, and people who attended the conference because they just wanted to learn the truth. You owe it to yourself to watch this docuseries. The path it will lead you down will change the way you think about everyday life.

I gave you the information about Chris Wark, who offered a great way to attack a cancer diagnosis. I'd also like to give you a list of other clinics that fight cancer with mostly natural approaches. These first three are in Mexico. Some of the treatments used are illegal in the United States for this reason or that, or non-FDA approval. But these are therapies that people want and search out, and they usually end up in Mexico to get them. One of the most commonly known therapies is B-17 injections, or Laetrile. You can get this treatment in an injection which ties in with other treatments as a form of integrative oncology.

Laetrile is found in some natural seeds, most commonly apricot seeds, and part of the compound is a natural form of cyanide which attacks cancer cells but does not harm normal cells.

Here is a list of the main clinics that I have learned about and from which I've heard the founders, experts, and doctors speak to their approaches.

In Mexico:

- Gerson Institute
- Hope 4 Cancer
- Hoxsey Biomedical Clinic

In the United States:

- Burzynski Clinic
- Exodus Health Center (Dr. Jockers)

Dr. Burzynski is another doctor I'd like to highlight. He discovered his own science-backed cancer treatment in the 1970's and is still using it today — antineoplaston therapy. There is a lot of controversy around this therapy and Dr. Burzynski has been in and out of court with the FDA and the Texas medical board for years. But he has had great responses and success stories with patients who had inoperable tumors. His therapy, in conjunction with others, has had success and is overall less toxic than chemotherapy alone. [7,8,9,10] As with any therapy, do your own research and decide what's right for you.

EPIGENETICS

The study of epigenetics has really come to the forefront of science in recent years. We are learning that genes can express themselves in different ways given the environment that they are exposed to.

Genes have switches that can be turned on or off, and these genes can be affected by the way you choose to live your life. They can be protective and preventative; the right food can talk to your genes and turn on protection for cells when undergoing chemo, while simultaneously turning off protection of the cancerous cells, thus enhancing the chemo effect. The genes can also be preventative in the same manner by protecting good cells and making the bad cells vulnerable to the immune system, thus preventing disease from ever forming.

A big topic with cancer is the genes. Do cancer genes run in the family? Did someone get cancer because they inherited the genes from the family? The most publicized genes for cancer are the BRCA1 and BRCA2. Women and men who have a mutation in this gene are more susceptible to cancer at an early age.[11]

Some of us are familiar with Angelina Jolie's story. She is just one of many who decided to have a preventative mastectomy after discovering that she had the BRCA mutation. A few years later, she had a blood test that showed markers for potential cancer growth; she then had her ovaries and fallopian tubes removed. She did not have a cancer diagnosis at the time but decided to take these measures based on the BRCA mutations. I don't know what her lifestyle was like, but how could you really blame her? She lost her mother and other close family members to these cancers, and I'm sure fear played a part in her decisions.[12]

An interesting study shows that BRCA-positive cancer patients may actually come out of treatment better off than those who are negative for the mutation.[13] Though BRCA2 mutation death rates become similar to those of non-carriers after longer amounts of time.[14] What if this gene mutation didn't predispose people to cancer in the first place?[15]

I hope this information can help someone who does have the BRCA mutation avoid becoming part of the 5-10% of the population that develops cancer. This discussion should help them take a deeper look, put the fear, uncertainty, and doubt (FUD) aside, and ask a lot of questions before coming to a rash decision about preventative measures. It's only you who can make this decision.

If I had the mutation, I would be asking questions like:

- Could the lifestyle I'm leading flip these genetic switches?

- Are there ways to live or foods to eat that can turn cancer cells off, or destroy them, and turn my immune system on?
- Is there a diet or way of eating that can talk to the DNA of my genes to prevent disease?

Diet is obviously a major factor in delivering the life nutrients and energy to the core of your cells, which enables them to flip. Also, environmental factors must be taken into consideration as well, like where you live and what environmental toxins you are being exposed to. If these toxins are overwhelming your body and not flushing out, especially at an early age, they could have a very negative impact on your epigenetics, as this 2017 study from the Journal of Clinical Epigenetics showed in Fresno California.[16] Ambient air pollutants cause DNA differences in asthma cases, in addition to other long-term effects of exposure to pollution-rich areas. "Prenatal ambient air pollutant exposure alters epigenetic programming" and "children are at greater risk of developing asthma when exposed to higher concentrations of AAPs", or ambient air pollutants.

Being aware of the unavoidable free radicals around you, and helping your body flush these toxins out, is a key preventative step in keeping your good genes switched on and bad genes switched off.

Diet can also play an integral part in controlling your genes. Coming back to our BRCA mutations examples, are there foods or actions that can help prevent these mutated BRCA genes from forming cancer, or repair the genes themselves? Could the extract of a Thai herb be chemo protective, or help repair the mutated strands of DNA that give the BRCA gene such high cancer risk? One study, "The effectiveness of cucurbitacin B in BRCAI defective breast cancer cells", out of Thailand suggests so.[17] Published in 2013 in PLOS One, Cucurbitacin B is a potential agent for long-term anticancer chemo prevention. Cucurbitacin is a terpene, which is the protective compound found in many plants or herbs and was found to be a "favorable phytochemical for cancer prevention".

This is a perfect example of how a natural plant can change the way genes express themselves. I'm not sure what this herb is, or if it's a digestible culinary herb, but the life force of this herb (cucurbitacin) was extracted, given to someone who had a negative gene expression, and assisted the person with whole body healing and prevention.

Our Thai herb example is great, but this is probably not a readily available therapy to most people; I doubt your family doctor has a vile on hand. But, what if there were common foods that anyone could get pretty much anywhere in the world? Eating these foods alone may not be enough to affect the expression of our genes, but could a mineral that's readily available in those foods be enough? Brazil nuts, eggs, mushrooms, cheese, oysters, sunflower seeds. These foods all contain selenium, with Brazil nuts serving as the best example. Six to eight nuts deliver 777% of our daily allowance.

A study from the American Association for Cancer Research, Cancer Epidemiology Biomarkers and Prevention, shows that the frequency of chromosome breakage in BRCAI genes was normalized after 3 months of oral selenium[18] intake and was similar to the examples of non-carriers of the BRCA mutations.

Now this is a great study and very good knowledge for BRCAI mutation holders to be aware of. What's even better is while this therapy could be treating a gene mutation, it could also be helping the body rid itself of heavy metals. Selenium is also a natural chelator, which means it binds to stubborn metals and helps flush or detox them out of the body. Selenium is a holistic therapy used to treat and prevent disease, and it doubles as a tool we can use toward whole body healing and prevention.

Let me introduce you to Thomas Seyfried. He is a professor of biology at Boston College. The science that he has been performing is pointing toward cancer not at all being a genetic disease, but a metabolic disease. This is a complete 180-degree turn from what is discussed above. He points to cancer being caused by sugars, glucose, and glutamine fermenting within cells and driving cancer growth. Many foods that the standard American diet (SAD) consists of turn into these fuels during digestion, unless they are sugar-filled foods to begin with. Sugar feeds cancer.

We will dive into Professor Seyfried's work later and see the amazing results that doctors have had using his thesis and therapies. According to Professor Seyfried, patients are coming out of treatment healthier than they were before, a far cry from people who are being burned, poisoned, and operated on to address the same disease. Some of his theses and therapies also cover the topic of epigenetics as well, including the therapies and diets that can control how our genes act.

Now, rounding out our look into epigenetics, we see that the environment and foods can play a major role in how our genes express themselves. Let's look at another wonder that has come to the surface that may be a very powerful preventative against cancer, as well as cardiovascular disease.

RESVERATROL

I s red wine good or bad to drink? Obviously, in excess, alcohol can take a toll, but resveratrol is the key compound that gives wine its health benefits. It is found in the skins of red grapes. And there are also other foods containing resveratrol, which is a protective plant compound made by these foods. For example, blueberries, and other dark berries, red wine, dark chocolate, knot weed extract, and pistachios are all power houses containing resveratrol.

There is a lot of science on the benefits of resveratrol, though skeptics insist that there have been no studies on humans regarding the benefits. This study from the BMC Journal of Nutrition shows that by eating grapes, the chances of colon cancer are reduced in a group of 30 people,[19] by suppressing a signaling pathway that is activated in 85% of colon cancer patients. Also, another study from the American Association for Cancer Research shows the presence of chemo-preventative properties after giving various dose ranges to mice, with the only side effect observed being gastrointestinal; however, the dosing was deemed safe.[20]

These are great studies, and there are many more like them. But the real significance is how resveratrol may protect against cancer, and at the same time may also have protective cardiovascular properties, too! Name a drug on the market that could potentially address the two biggest killers in the United States today. The science is pointing in this direction, so why isn't this plastered all over the news?

Getting back to the cardiovascular study: resveratrol therapy was given to rodents who had been exposed to cigarette smoke. The results were anti-inflammatory and reduced oxidative stress.[21] Taken together, the key word in both of those outcomes is anti-aging. This is all from a compound derived from red grapes, knot weed, and dark berries. Folks, this is a two-for-one if there ever was one. Imagine the prevention that can take place if you were ingesting resveratrol while living a healthy lifestyle?! Preventative anti-aging? Yes, please!

I have heard resveratrol mentioned several times while listening to speakers or reading articles about the health benefits of red wine and the skins of dark berries. I always have this information in mind when consuming them, but one anti-aging authority really emphasized the powers of resveratrol and intrigued me to take a closer look – Naomi Whittel. Naomi has been helping women lose weight, control hormones, and anti-age. Many other benefits have come out of her research and life experiences, and they are all explained in her book *Glow15*, a book I have bought for more women than I can count on both hands. Even though this book is tailored toward women -- I'm a guy in case you didn't know – I've read it and I'm following her practices as well. Look her up!

ESSENTIAL OILS

I mentioned earlier about how it is possible to support yourself if you are already undergoing chemotherapy or radiation. Take these examples to heart, talk to your oncologist about them, and ask them hard questions before they just say no, because they will, because they don't want to be bothered. But this is your life, and maybe that could be the question for them. Is supporting myself through these therapies that we both know are toxic a bother to you? Is my life a bother to you?

In my book, essential oils are medicine. They can be inhaled, ingested, or used topically. They are the epitome of treatment and prevention. You don't have to look far to come up with that conclusion. Plants are medicine, and every religion and culture in the world has been distilling plants for their medicinal properties for at least 5,000 years. If you are religious, the Bible has around 300 references to them. The three Wise Men brought Frankincense and Myrrh as their gifts to the baby Jesus. Another gift was gold, although some believe that it was turmeric.

If you only believe what science concludes, there are 17,000 studies on essential oils referenced on PubMed, an archive of biomedical and life science journal literature. Essential oils are very potent and very strong. They are concentrated forms of plant matter. Use caution or advise with a naturopath or an essential oil coach like myself (currently enrolled in an essential oil coaching school accredited by the American Association of Drugless Practitioners) before applying, ingesting, or inhaling. Always avoid applying oils to sensitive areas, sensitive skin, and eyes. Some oils, like grapefruit, can cause prescribed medications to work improperly. Always consult a professional or educate yourself before using essential oils.

I personally use essential oils every day for various reasons. I have them at home and even in the office and offer them to people who have ailments. One of my co-workers has bad bouts of asthma. She has a huge inhaler, and sometimes asks me to make her some *medicina*. I mix peppermint, holy basil, eucalyptus, and lemongrass in a coffee cup, and then pour a little scalding water over the oil. She inhales the steam vapors through her nose and mouth, and it opens her airways, giving her instant relief. I mix the same blend with a carrier oil like coconut, and she rubs it on her chest to keep inhaling the fumes while she works. This also gives the oils a chance to seep into her chest to aid her. And again, with the same combination of oils (one drop of each), some coconut oil, and a touch of honey, she can ingest this mix throughout the day. She has told me numerous times that the medicine I make is far better than what is prescribed to her by her doctor.

The compounds of these oils are so micro that they can get through tight dense areas and can breach the blood brain barrier to deliver these compounds to your brain, and I'm sure that they could seep into your chest cavity as well. I have felt an oil like peppermint give that burn deep into my chest – the kind of burn you would feel from Icy Hot.

These essential oils can also be used for something as simple as a household cleaner, or even insect spray like I make when the boys and I go camping: apple cider vinegar, vodka, lemongrass, eucalyptus, tea tree, and peppermint. We all ditched the toxic store-bought spray and didn't get bitten once!

Once you start using essential oils, you start swapping out your medicine cabinet. All the sugary cough syrups and lozenges are in the trash. Commercial toothpaste with fluoride is a thing of the past; I either use salts with essential oils and neem, or a natural toothpaste with a few drops of oils added on top. Commercial lotions that contain toxic substances have been replaced with homemade essential oil lotions that are free of toxins. They smell much better, and these moisturizers can also fight cancer while absorbing through your skin and being inhaled through the nose and mouth.

The king of essential oils is Frankincense, which is distilled from the sap of the Boswellia tree. It is referenced around 150 times in the Bible. The long list of benefits includes relaxing the brain, relieving anxiety, aiding depression and mood disorders, and controlling alcoholism. Also, anti-inflammation, immune support, and meditation assistance are among its benefits. This oil can really bring a sense of peacefulness and overall well-being.

There are also studies pointing to the benefits of Frankincense treating cancer and/or preventing it. Pancreatic cancer is one of the worst, with a five-year survival rate. (Five years is the benchmark of a long-term survivor). A study showed that Frankincense can have an apoptotic effect, or cell death on pancreatic adenocarcinoma cells, giving it a potentially good use case as an alternative treatment against pancreatic cancer.[22]

Another study shows that a blend of essential oils may be used to combat breast cancer.

Science out of China suggests that Frankincense, pine needle, and geranium essential oils could have antitumor affects. They could also be a good alternative to therapies where toxicity and chemo-resistance are causes for failure. These oils may contribute to apoptosis (cell death), are anti-bacterial, anti-fungal, and possess anti-cancer activity. Further studies are needed to strengthen this case.[23]

This preventative ability is further demonstrated by science out of Italy. Frankincense has been used for thousands of years in Ayurvedic medicine and is known to regulate inflammation, oxidative stress, and immune dysregulation.[24] However, one statement mentioned in these studies brings up a key factor in essential oil use. Cautions should be exercised when buying these oils as there are a lot of inferior oils out there on the market. Commercial oils are probably like most commercial products, mass produced with little quality. Look for organic oils, or oils that are rated "food grade".

Hopefully one day, we will see frankincense on the market in the form of a supplement. I think people are waking up to the fact and starting to support these oils as medicine. With regards to frankincense, the sap from a tree is truly a medicine, as are all plants.[25] As you can see, one essential oil can have multiple benefits, and all of these oils act the same way. While using an oil for one purpose, you are also preventing in multiple other ways.

Who are the authorities on essential oils? Dr. Josh Axe and Dr. Eric Zielinski.

Dr. Axe runs the essential oil coaching school that I'm enrolled in. After a first diagnosis and conventional treatment, he used essential oils as a weapon in conjunction with other protocols to cure his own mother of cancer.

SUPPORTING CHEMO WITH ESSENTIAL OILS

I f you opt for chemotherapy as your cancer treatment, there are ways to support your immune system while it undergoes this great assault. Chemo is good at one thing – killing cells. Most chemo treatments do not target the cancer cells; they can kill any cell, good or bad. As an alternative, let's explore some additional examples of natural treatments that double as preventatives.

Next is another great example of how frankincense could be used to replace a drug that has many known bad side effects. Brain tumors can cause swelling, or cerebral edema. Dexamethasone is a drug that is used to keep that swelling down and to relieve nausea from chemotherapy. The side effects of dexamethasone can be depression, hyperthyroidism, and even diabetes. It's also been shown to damage the mitochondria of cells, create oxidative stress and cell death, and in treatment with newborns, it can affect neurological function.

In a placebo-controlled, double blind study, 14 patients were given boswellic acid, the active compound in frankincense, and 13 patients were given a placebo. The results supported that boswellic acid can indeed alleviate swelling in the brain caused by tumors.[26] This evidence points to natural plant matter doing the same job as a pharmaceutical drug, minus the dangerous side effects. Why is this not plastered on the 10 o'clock news?

Next time you bang your head on the counter, will you take an aspirin or maybe rub in some frankincense oil? I personally would go for the frankincense, but if you do hit your head and you see stars, or have a ringing in your ear, please go to the emergency room and get checked out. These are signs of a concussion. Frankincense can help alleviate swelling, so apply it on the way, but by no means would I rely on it to treat an acute trauma.

Let's give dexamethasone some more natural competition, with no side effects. I mentioned above that it was also administered to relieve nausea. Peppermint essential oil has the same effects. I don't know how much dexamethasone costs, but I do know that two ounces of organic peppermint essential oil probably costs $30 or so. A 2013 article from the European Institute of Oncology showed a randomized double-blind clinical trial in which peppermint essential oil reduced the nausea and vomiting of patients who'd undergone chemotherapy, and served as a very cost-effective alternative to dexamethasone.[27] Natural plant matter is relieving symptoms just as effectively as toxic drugs. I'm going to go out on a limb here, but if there were or are other studies using peppermint for hangovers and car sickness, I'm sure it would aid in the relief of these as well.

SUPPORTING CHEMO WITH MEDICINAL MUSHROOMS

Fungus has been given a bad name, and most people really think that fungus or mold need to be killed. Now there are harmful funguses like black mold in the walls of your house, or fungal infections like Valley Fever, which may have taken the life of my father. But as we will see in this section, fungus can do amazing things as well. Fungus will be the first on site to rebuild a damaged ecosystem, like a decimated forest. It may be misunderstood, but fungus is the first on the scene when things are depleted or malnourished. It is there to clean up, detox the environment, and start decomposition to allow new life to begin again.

Now let's look at something you may be surprised by. (Well, I hope this isn't the first surprise you have come across in this reading!) Mushrooms! Medicinal mushrooms. Let's see how fungus can aid your body in areas where there is malnourishment or disease. Could they support you and your immune system while undergoing chemotherapy? Here we go again!

The Chaga mushroom is found in the northern hemisphere and mostly grows on dead birch trees. Can this fungus help rebuild damaged bone marrow because of chemo? Mice were given an immune-suppressing substance and then treated with Chaga extract, and the science here supports strong immune-enhancing qualities while undergoing chemo.[28]

It's very interesting to read a study with the big scientific terms and words that us laypeople will have to look up, but then, just when your eyes are about to glaze over the words, "wild mushrooms" pop up. Sometimes cancer cells can become resistant to treatment, which is not something you want to hear after going through rounds of chemo.

Yes, wild mushrooms that contain verticillin were shown to weaken chemo-resistant colon cancer cells and aid in the process of apoptosis — cell death. Now this is not to say that stopping by the farmers market and buying some mushrooms to sauté is going to cure your colon cancer, but the study showed how safe doses of verticillin affected genes and killed cancer cells. Fluorouracil 5 is the standard chemotherapy for high risk, high stage colorectal cancer patients. Though it is very common for patients to become chemo-resistant to this therapy, the study "Epigenetic-based therapy to overcome human colon cancer Fluorouracil 5 resistance" shows that verticillin can have the same effects as the chemo drugs.[29]

I have to give you one more because it's one of the most basic things I have ever seen, and I guarantee that nobody would ever put these words in the same sentence. White button mushrooms and prostate cancer. Now maybe these exotic Chaga, Reishi, or Cordycepe mushrooms from some faraway place could have medicinal properties; eastern medicine could really have something there, but plain old white button mushrooms?

You may have heard that a common test for prostate cancer is a PSA, or prostate-specific antigen, test. In a phase I trial, white button mushroom powder was the therapy given to a group. Various results occurred, but the overall PSA counts went down, and some went to undetectable levels. Also, recurring prostate cancer was affected by the decrease in immune system suppression.[30]

Have I driven the point home? Have I pounded the table enough to look at food and the properties in them as ways to treat and prevent disease? The sap of trees, wild mushrooms, dark berries, brazil nuts, distilled oils of plants, herbs, spices. But what about something so simple, a treatment you can use anytime, anywhere? And here is the kicker, it takes up no time, it costs nothing, and the list of benefits is a whole other book. Too good to be true?

FASTING. AUTOPHAGY. ANTI-AGING

We live in a world of consumption and corporations. The corporations are constantly advertising to consume their products. That's business. But most of these businesses don't have your best interest at heart. Food is in our face 24/7: it's easily accessible and we have been taught or programmed that we need to eat constantly. Even some gym trainers or health field professionals encourage dieters to eat more small meals throughout the day. What needs to be understood is it takes a lot of energy for the body to digest food. We are either in a rest and restore phase, or digesting.

When we are in a constant digestive phase, we never give the body a chance to rest and repair. Eating all the time, and especially eating late or eating right before going to sleep can be a very bad habit. Let's look at eating right before bed. We have all spent time on the treadmill or elliptical and have seen how much work it takes to burn a few calories. It's the same in the body. Our body is working overtime to digest food to give us energy, but this shouldn't happen when we are in a sleep state. We don't need that energy while we are sleeping. It's taking away our time to heal. Not allowing the body to repair itself can turn into a dangerous situation, especially if the food you are eating is not good quality.

Valter Longo, PhD, is a biologist who heads the University of Southern California's Longevity Institute. Anti-aging is a big part of his work. He has found that in our Western societies, where we are constantly consuming poor-quality food, we've really put a damper on a process called autophagy.

The subject of autophagy, by the way, won the Nobel Prize in medicine in 2016 with a paper from Yoshinori Ohsumi. Autophagy translates to self-eating. This occurs when a damaged or improperly functioning cell is self-consumed and then replaced with new cells. Stem cells are activated when fasting, a process that also produces new cells and regeneration. When we are in a fasting state, our cells can flip on the autophagy switch. This process is very beneficial for anti-aging and general prevention.

Think about that – by not eating, we give our body the chance to repair improperly functioning cells, and not let them disrupt the energies of other cells. That's anti-aging *and* prevention. Let's get into Dr. Longo's science on fasting and the countless number of benefits and preventatives that go along with it, and also cover his first-ever meal plan that gives you all the benefits of fasting, while you are actually eating.

As it pertains to cancer, Dr. Longo and a host of others conducted a study where the subjects fasted 24, 48 and 72 hours prior to receiving chemotherapy. Insulin growth factors and properties were measured as markers to the effect of the fasting. In the end, fasting was deemed safe for cancer patients around the times of chemotherapy administration.[31]

Essentially, fasting can add a layer of protection to normal cells as they are in a stressed state from not being fueled and can protect themselves against the chemotherapy. Whereas the cancer cells are being deprived and are opened or unprotected and exposed to the toxins of chemo, enhancing this therapy.

Our whipping boy is back in our studies. Dexamethasone, as we know, is given to a lot of cancer patients, and it increases glucose levels. But wait, glucose is sugar and sugar feeds cancer, yes? Then why is it used? I don't know. But this study on mice shows that fasting can regulate glucose levels or hyperglycemia, and the effects can be reversed.[32]

So we now see how fasting is another way to assist your body through the negative effects of chemo and toxic drugs. It's a way to fight cancer cell growth by starving the cancer of the sugar it needs, which can also be a great preventative by never allowing cancer cells a chance to grow in the first place. Fasting: it's free, and it's been used by civilizations and religions for thousands of years. Who knew that not eating could be so beneficial?

Above, I mentioned Dr. Longo's fasting diet. He has created a program where you eat a minimal number of calories and the body still thinks it's in a fasting state.[33] I have personally completed this diet, and I did it at the perfect time after some extensive travel where I let my diet get away from me. Hey, I'm a chef and it was always a dream of mine to wander the streets of Thailand and Vietnam and enjoy the street food. But that's another book. And no, I didn't get sick once, probably because my immune system was so strong after following everything I've been writing about.

So back to the diet that "mimics" fasting. I followed the very easy instructions, ate the tasty plant-based food provided, and felt great. I also noticed the slimming of my waist, where the eight pounds of stored fat melted away. That was the physical outcome of the program, which is great but not the main reason I tried it. The real magic was what was happening inside my body. Cell regeneration, autophagy, and probably the easiest preventative measure I have ever taken against disease. Now let's look at the actual study where there are some serious claims.[34] Cancer, cardiovascular disease, diabetes, and aging. The risk for all of these conditions can be decreased and prevented by using this powerful tool, fasting, or a diet that mimics it. Thank you Dr. Longo!!

While on this program, I was very active about it on social media, and there were quite a few people who tried it after they saw me posting about it. But literally a few minutes ago as I was reviewing this part of my writing, I received a text from a fellow health coach who said she had just come off the diet. Synchronicity!! She was down six pounds, which was great, but she knew she was preventing issues that run genetically in her family. We know about epigenetics, we know that a diet or lifestyle like this is the best way you can prevent diseases that may run in the family.

What led Dr. Longo to create this diet for individuals was a fast-mimicking diet for cancer patients. This diet would need to be under a doctor's supervision, but the same principles apply and we have seen the science to back it up.

I encourage you to check out this diet by using the last two citations (33,34): Prolon's Fasting Mimicking Diet and the study "A periodic diet that mimics fasting promotes multi-system regeneration," out of Cell Metabolism from 2015. I know most people immediately are turned off by the word *fasting*. The thought of skipping a meal, the thought of feeling hungry. There are many ways to fast and most people do some sort of intermittent fasting just by getting a good night's sleep. Would you give fasting a shot if you knew that you could start to prevent three major diseases that are plaguing America today?

Do I need to even ask this question?

Who are the experts on fasting and longevity? Obviously, Dr. Longo, but also Naomi Whittel, who has a Facebook group that provides support for people who are committing themselves to five days of water fasting. I myself haven't had the courage to try this yet, but I have been sticking with Dr. Longo's program of the fast mimicking diet.

Another expert that I have heard speak is Dr. Edward Group III. He has taken water fasting to over two weeks and has given examples of people having godly experiences or even fasting for up to 40 days. I believe he is writing a book devoted to water fasting. He also covers some great myths people fear when they hear the word *fasting*. One such fear is, "I will lose muscle mass." Actually, fasting increases HGH (human growth hormone) levels, maintaining muscle mass. After glucose or sugar stores are burned for energy, the body will start breaking down stored fat and the liver will start producing ketones to feed the brain and body. If your total body fat falls below 5%, then you will be in danger of muscle-wasting. That is the time cortisol will be produced and muscles will start to be torn down and turned into glucose.

Tying this together, people are also afraid they will starve to death or their blood sugars will fall too low. Yes, your blood sugar will fall, but when glucose is depleted, your body will use fat for energy. If you were on a high carbohydrate diet that digests lots of glucose and have never allowed your body to use fat as a fuel, you may feel some adverse effects, but when the brain becomes adapted to receiving ketones as a fuel, you will start to see a clarity you may have not experienced before, or the godly experiences. Here is a 2007 hypothesis out of Science Direct that can maybe further explain this godly feeling or feeling of euphoria.[35] Ketone bodies are produced when a ketogenic diet is followed. Beta-hydroxybutyrate (BHB) and gamma-hydroxybutyrate (GHB) are produced as part of these ketone bodies and the combination of the two on the brain may give the mild feeling of euphoria.

Water-only fasting for extended periods should be done under medical supervision. Going at it alone for extended periods can be dangerous. There are lots of centers around the world that you can go to for supervised fasts. If you are thinking this may be something that may help heal a condition, do a lot of research and make sure the clinic is top-notch and has a good reputation. I've heard stories of people going to some of these detox centers and almost dying. On the other hand, I have come across a few that look to be reputable and are helping people every day in a safe way. Here are a couple:

- True North Health Center in Santa Rosa California
- Hippocrates Health Center in West Palm Beach Florida

Now I have given numerous examples of whole body healing and prevention throughout this book. Two of my favorite impactful topics have been fasting and resveratrol. They both address the two major diseases and killers in the world to-date. In a 2010 study from Cell Death and Disease, scientists conclude that autophagy is required to prolong life and slow the effects of aging, and two ways to get there are calorie restriction or fasting and resveratrol. Another cool study I couldn't leave out, since it covers whole body healing, prevention and anti-aging.

Its 1:30 p.m. I'm going to break my 16-hour fast and have some blueberries, pistachios, and coco nibs, our resveratrol rich foods![36]

Hopefully you now realize how fasting is very beneficial. Throughout this discussion I mentioned a few new terms with which you may or may not be familiar. I want to focus on one in particular. I'm sure you have heard it: ketones, or ketogenic diet. Intermittent fasting and a ketogenic diet go hand-in-hand, and they are the perfect complement to one another.

WHAT IS THE KETOGENIC DIET?

The ketogenic diet is a high fat, moderate protein, low carbohydrate diet. When this diet is followed properly, your body will enter a state of ketosis. This is when your body has run low or run out of glucose (sugars) to burn for energy. After this happens, the body will tap into either fat stores or use recently consumed fats for energy. The fats are broken down, and then ketones are produced by the liver and used to fuel the brain and body. Ketones are your body's preferred fuel source and are used in a much more efficient way. Ketones are a cleaner form of energy compared to sugars.

At birth, we were all once fat burners, but with the rise of carbohydrate consumption from misinformation like the old government food pyramid, which suggested carbs as the main foundation of meals, our bodies have adapted to using sugars as our primary fuel source. You can see how burning sugar can be problematic; we know that cancer feeds on sugar, and that sugars can cause insulin resistance, leading to diabetes.

DON'T EAT DOUGHNUTS

This is something I don't think most people ask themselves when they eat a meal. What will this food turn into as it's being digested? Foods made of refined carbs, like breads, pasta, white rice, and baked sweets, will turn into sugar in the body. When following a keto diet, you are much more prone to asking yourself this question. Take a doughnut for example. It's a triple threat. It's made with refined flour that will turn into sugar. It could be even worse if the flour was made from genetically modified wheat. (We'll get into that.) It's made with sugar, probably in the dough itself, then the glaze, sugar topping, or filling. Then it's fried, most likely in an oil that will cause oxidative stress. Just skip it!

Currently the ketogenic diet is in "fad" territory. A lot of people are jumping onboard and most of them are following the diet wrong. But this way of living and eating is nowhere near a fad. I've heard doctors use the term therapeutic ketosis. The ketogenic diet has absolutely been used to help treat major health conditions. As always, there are skeptics

I've encountered and there are those who don't follow the diet properly.

Here is where the skeptics come in. A high-fat diet? Doesn't fat make you fat? Won't fat clog your arteries and give you heart disease? Kind of like our previous example of how we are programmed (if you will) to constantly eat. We have been programmed to think that fat is the enemy, that fat will make you fat, that fat will clog your arteries. I'd like to point to a meta-analysis of 21 studies that was performed. After five to 23 years of follow-up of some 350,000 people, it was concluded that coronary heart disease or cardiovascular disease was not associated with saturated fat.[37]

Yes, there are some fats that are absolutely the enemy. And yes, consuming high amounts of fats along with a high carb diet can be dangerous, but when talking about a keto diet done the proper way, the fats consumed are healthy and of high quality. Let's look at some proof.

A study looked at chronic obstructive pulmonary disease, which is a lung issue where patients have a hard time breathing. Groups were given low-carb, high-fat and high-carb, low-fat diets. The conclusion was that pulmonary function can be improved when following a high fat low carb diet.[38] I know this is not about arteries, but nonetheless, pathways were cleared for these patients to breathe easier by changing their diet to ketogenic.

Let's address the notion that fats that are bad for you. Of course, these would be manmade fats. Omega-6 fats like vegetable oils, corn oil, cotton seed oil, grapeseed oil, peanut oil, and canola oil. These are all very unstable fats and when heated for cooking or frying (our doughnut), it will denature the oils, and cause them to oxidize. Some of these oils oxidize just sitting on the shelf at the local market. When an oxidized oil is ingested, it then causes oxidative stress in the body, and this in turn can cause inflammation in your arteries, gut, and elsewhere. Oxidative stress is like your body rusting on the inside. This causes inflammation in your arteries and intestines, and when you are in a state of chronic inflammation, health issues can arise down the road. It's important to know what's in your food: these oils are everywhere, they're sneaky, and used in abundance. One of the big offenders is salad dressing. Read labels, folks!

A speaker (whose name unfortunately escapes me) once gave an example of a certain well-known health food store and the prepared food sections. You know, where the food is sitting over a steam table and you help yourself. If you ask what the ingredients are, you will find that they use canola oil; yes, it's non-GMO; yes, it's organic, etc. But these foods have been sitting out at an elevated temperature for hours. It doesn't matter how organic the food is: it's being served with oxidized oils that are absolutely going to cause oxidative stress and inflammation in your body.

What are the fats you should be consuming on a keto diet? Healthy HDL-promoting fats, first-pressed organic coconut oil, biodynamic or organic olive oils, grass-fed butter or ghee (clarified butter), avocado oil, organic nut oils, pistachios, macadamia nuts and their oils, wild caught, high-quality salmon products from Alaska, and avocados. Don't be afraid of other saturated fats in moderation like from grass-fed beef products, and keep the skin on your organic chicken, or get the fat nice and crispy on your pasture-raised, walnut-finished pork chops. Sorry, I'm a chef, I get excited.

Now let's move into animal products and animal fats. Animal protein and fat can be a part of the ketogenic diet, but the key here is the quality and amount consumed. I would like to reinforce that a ketogenic diet is not a high protein diet. Consuming too much animal protein will digest into glucose and can take away the effects of the diet or pop you out of ketosis. This is probably the most common mistake I see people make. They think that it's okay to eat animal fat, so it's okay to eat bacon, and steak, and pork, and other fatty delicious meats. But as I said, this is not a high-protein diet. I eat meat and fish, but only on occasion; I like to follow more of a plant-based keto diet where I'm getting my carbs and protein from plant-based foods. Obviously, this will appeal to vegetarians and vegans, by eating your protein and carbs from plant sources or cruciferous vegetables, like kale, broccoli, Brussels sprouts, spinach, cauliflower, collard greens, and swiss chard. Hemp seeds are packed with protein and are so much easier to digest than animal protein.

Back to our animal products: quality is of the utmost importance. If buying bacon, look for uncured, or bacon that's doesn't contain nitrates or nitrites (carcinogens). Same with deli meats or other processed meat products. By the way, you are probably best avoiding these processed foods.

EAT REAL WHOLE FOODS!

R ead labels and look for sugar and other additives that will affect your carb intake or are unhealthy. Look for animal products, like beef, pork, chicken, and lamb, that come from local small farms where they are free range, pasture-raised, organic, or grass fed with no hormones or antibiotics. Meat products that are commercial or mass-produced are foods you do not want to be consuming.

Fish is also another caution. There are a lot of farmed fish varieties out there that are fed corn-based, soy-based, grain-based, GMO-laden feed, and like all mass-produced, mass-raised animals, they are stuffed into small confined prison-like conditions where disease can spread throughout.

The prize fish for a keto diet would have to be a wild, line-caught option like Alaskan Salmon, Coho, or King. The fillet and roe from these fish are packed with omega-3's and are a great source of healthy fat that fit right into keto. Others would be anchovy, mackerel, sardines, trout, or fattier fish that are line-caught from rivers, lakes, or streams. Be diligent about the fish you are buying, and make sure it was caught sustainably. Where was it caught? What are the waters like where the fish is coming from? I'm concerned about the whole Pacific Ocean after the Fukushima disaster in Japan in 2011. To this day, the radiation has not been contained and the waste is still flowing into the ocean. Mercury levels are another concern. People seem to be consuming a lot of tuna in popular sushi and now-trending poke. Tuna, swordfish, tilefish, and sturgeon all contain high amounts of mercury. These are fish that can get quite big and old as they grow, and when they are exposed to more toxins, the greater the probability that humans will ingest them.

I'd like to give a plug here and suggest people check out Vital Seafood in Alaska. They sell prized salmon and salmon products and are a very reputable company. I've become a customer and, as a chef, I am using their products every day in my kitchen. Their salmon oils are probably the best out there as the process starts right on the boat just hours after the fish has been caught. Also, these oils are the best source of omega-3's from the freshest waters and sustainably sourced fish.

Let's switch gears and reflect on a statement I made above about therapeutic ketosis.

In particular, let's zero in on the work of Professor Seyfried of Boston College. It is enthralling to listen to Professor Seyfried speak. To some he may be controversial, but all his research is backed by his science that is executed with others. His results are also backed by the doctors who are implementing his techniques in the treatment of patients. I heard Professor Seyfried speak at The Truth about Cancer conference in Orlando, held by cancer researcher and expert

Ty Bollinger and his wife Charlene. The following citations are straight from his presentation and his own science.

The bold claim is: cancer is not a genetic disease, but a metabolic disease. This goes against what almost every medical professional is taught about cancer.[39] Breaking his thesis down to a cellular level by looking at the science provided concludes that the damage, or mutations in cells, is first started in the mitochondria of the cell. The mutations then proceed to the nucleus of the cell. The mitochondria are the metabolism or energy of the cell, and the nucleus is the genome or genetics of the cell. The normal thinking and basis of a lot of research is the opposite – the damage starts in the nucleus from genetics then proceeds to the rest of the cell.[40]

Go ahead and read that again.

It's the perfect study of epigenetics, the environment inside the cell is causing mutations or damage to the genetic aspect of the cell. The mutations, according to Professor Seyfried or the Warburg theory, are being caused by damages to cell respiration.[41] This damage is caused by glucose or glutamine fermenting in the cell. The cells don't respire the available oxygen; it instead ferments it.

How can the mitochondria or the environment in which the nucleus lives adapt to affect the nucleus in a good way? Professor Seyfried explains that "depriving" the cells of glucose or sugars or "fermentable fuel" will give the cell the ability to respire the oxygen normally. What is the fuel that has this capability? Ketones! This means adapting a ketogenic diet, as ketones are a non-fermentable fuel.

There is more to the therapy than just a ketogenic diet, and like all therapies, there is no silver bullet. Each treatment needs to be customized to the individual. But by cutting out the fuel that is promoting the cancer growth, the diet can slow or stop the progression of the tumor or spread (metastasis) of cancer elsewhere.[42]

In a 1995 study out of Case Western Reserve University, School of Medicine in Cleveland, Ohio two female children who both had recurring inoperable brain tumors went through the standard of care. They were put on ketogenic diets and were able to stabilize the tumor growth. Scans showed glucose at the site of the tumors decreased. One girl went another 12 months on the diet and the tumors did not progress.[43]

Our whipping boy, dexamethasone, is back. As we know, it's given to prevent swelling and promotes glucose levels. Glioblastoma (brain tumor) patients are given dexamethasone and also undergo brain swelling radiation to combat these difficult tumors. When the brain swells under radiation, it also causes hyperglycemia (excess glucose in the blood). This shows that the standard of care that is most likely being prescribed by any standard oncologist is giving the tumor the exact fuel that it needs to grow.

The technique of starving cancer cells of the fuel that they need to survive and multiply starts with a ketogenic diet. This opens the cancer cells to other forms of treatments, while healthy cells develop a layer of protection. This therapy was given the name "press-pulse," and as Professor Seyfried and others show, press-pulse can be executed with no toxicity to the patient even with the use of some drugs and procedures.[44] Professor Seyfried states that "patients leave the therapy healthier than when they started." Now you may say that these patients had cancer, that they were not healthy. Yes, this is a valid point, but if you look at patients who went through conventional treatments, they usually come out with a host of other problems from the toxic therapies. Here is an observational study from 2017 out of Cureus. A single woman in a dire situation of triple negative breast cancer that spread to the liver and lymph nodes. I'm not sure if the therapy was press-pulse, but the outcome was significant.[45] After a 6-month protocol of a ketogenic diet, hyperbolic oxygen therapy, hyperthermia, and metabolically supported chemotherapy, the patient showed complete response.

We have looked at some pretty serious results using a ketogenic diet. Another that is worth pointing out is epilepsy. There are several studies pointing to the benefits of a keto diet, including how it intervenes in seizure activity. One study, The ketogenic diet: a 3- to 6-year follow-up of 150 children, out of Johns Hopkins, followed these children on the ketogenic diet for six years. Some percentage (in the high teens) were free of seizures, which is remarkable, but the diet also helped with reduction or discontinuance of medications. The outcome of getting off meds that caused all the side effects is an awesome feat, especially after only changing the diet of these children.[46] Not only was there a reduction in medications, but the ketogenic diet was also keeping children out of emergency rooms as well.[47]

I will mention this now and we will touch on it later. Medical marijuana products have also had great success at treating epilepsy. I have heard of cases of using one or the other, where they don't work for every patient. It raises the question of what the results could be if they were combined.

CARDIOVASCULAR

'm starting to see studies that examine cardioprotective features of a ketogenic diet. Rats that had decreased blood flow were given a ketogenic diet and a standard high carb diet; they were given this diet for 19 weeks and the outcome was cardioprotective.[48] So, let's keep looking into cardiovascular health. We know high cholesterol is associated with cardiovascular disease, but is it in the way that we think? Is cholesterol the bad guy that is causing this epidemic in America?

I want to share a story with you that I heard on Naomi Whittel's docuseries, *The Real Skinny on Fat*. She interviewed some experts on heart health, one being Dr. Steve Gundry. Dr. Gundry shared the story of a famous heart surgeon named Dr. Michael DeBakey. Dr. DeBakey was known to show up to meetings and for lunch having a big slice of triple cream brie cheese. This went against everything that cardiovascular surgeons believed in. "Doc, all that fat is going to kill you or clog your arteries." He would look at them and say, "it's not the fat."

Dr. DeBakey had a hypothesis. Cholesterol was not the cause of heart disease but was associated with it because it was always at "the scene of the accident." The actual cause of heart disease was inflammation, and the inflammation was being caused by eating the wrong kinds of carbohydrates. When these carbs are eaten and enter the bloodstream, they are looked at as a foreign substance by our immune system. White blood cells then attack the lining of blood vessels to get the intruder out, causing inflammation. It's essentially a battle taking place and the cleanup crew is cholesterol. Cholesterol is always at the site of the battle and when the blood vessels are inflamed, blockages occur.

Another shared observation from heart surgeons is about most new heart attack cases, where the patient is usually on a class of medication called statin. Statins are prescribed to lower cholesterol to avoid heart disease. This is usually prescribed when patients have elevated LDL levels. The statin corrects the issue of these levels, but most likely the patient is listening to the standard dietary recommendations and is following a low-fat, high-carb diet. This diet elevates triglyceride levels in the blood, which is the vehicle of moving sugars through the bloodstream. Conventionally, these lower LDL counts are a good thing, but they are almost artificially lowered due to the number of triglycerides still present. Now the bad part is that with the diet they are following, the HDL (good fats) count is very low. The patients are not eating enough good fats (HDL fats) that can go through and clean out blood vessels.

"The only purpose of food is to get olive oil into your mouth"
- Steven Gundry

Now why is the food pyramid upside down? Why were fats demonized? It could come down to Ancel Keys, a physiologist who did a flawed around-the-world study in the late 1950's looking at diets of different nations and, in the process, pretty much convinced the American Heart Association that dietary fat was the cause of cardiovascular heart disease. This was around the time Dwight Eisenhower suffered a heart attack while president. It seems everyone wanted something to blame, and there was cholesterol. Here we are today – most people still follow those guidelines and heart disease is the number one killer in the U.S.

The food pyramid has morphed into a "make a healthy plate" guide. Has our health become any better? Vegetables look to be the biggest portion, but it is about equal to the other three slices of the plate: grains, fruit, and protein, with a glass a dairy on the side. If you look at choosemyplate.gov, you'll see that low fat is still recommended for dairy, and even soy milk is considered a dairy now. The oils section is particularly interesting because there is no guidance on what good or bad oil is, apart from avoiding trans fats, thank God. All oils are lumped together, vegetable oil next to olive oil. Are these two oils equal?

Grains are separated into whole and refined, and it is stated that there are not enough whole grains consumed. Males ages 14-30 are recommended to eat eight ounces of grains which is equal to eight slices of bread per day. Women are recommended to eat six ounces.

Have these new dietary guidelines for the U.S. improved our health? Look at all the benefits of the ketogenic diet: a low-carb, moderate protein, high-good-fat diet, and then look at the "myplate" guidelines. As I mentioned, cardiovascular disease is still the number one killer today. The "myplate" guidelines started in 2011. In other words, eat real whole foods!

We can see where the root cause of this serious killer, heart disease, is coming from: our own government! Whether the foods recommended are subsidized and a part of the "big food" industry, they are obviously affecting the health of Americans in a negative way. This scenario is also playing into the hands of "big pharma," who, when all of these people start to develop health issues, begin to sell them their drugs. It's a perfect storm for corporations. Is it a coincidental storm or all by design? That's up to you. And for another book.

Let's look at some science related to heart disease and the drugs that are prescribed. We have touched on statins. This study states that high cholesterol in the elderly loses its correlation to heart disease and mortality, but these drugs are still prescribed, offering more risk than reward. The adverse effects can be cancer, neurodegenerative conditions, heart failure, and accelerated aging.[49]

Here is a study that may explain why statins have such side effects. We touched on the importance of selenium, the protective features and chelating effects it can have; well you may need to double or triple down if you are taking a statin.[50]

I have seen many studies and reviews that link things like sugar-sweetened beverages, hydrogenated trans oils, and even meat to heart disease. I don't feel the need to cite them as it's clear the effects these items have on our cardiovascular system. But what about something like aspirin? People take it all the time – a low dose of baby aspirin to prevent a cardiac event. But when people take it as a preventative, do the risks outweigh the benefits?

It has been shown that long-term low aspirin dosing may double the likelihood of gastrointestinal hemorrhaging.[51]

What are we going to do about this epidemic? As we previously covered, we need to pay attention to what we cover our plates with. We know a ketogenic diet that is full of healthy fats and lower protein is going to address issues of high cholesterol, and introducing foods high in resveratrol can also help prevent this disease. Very important to our overall health is vitamin D, but as research shows, it is also cardioprotective, and low vitamin D levels are associated with all-cause mortality.[52] How about one of the most preventative measures any of us can take to keep ourselves healthy and help prevent a lot of disease? Exercise. This study calls exercise a polypill or a prescription to prevent prevalent chronic conditions, like metabolism-related disorders, cancer, Alzheimer's, and cardiovascular disease. It doesn't get any more holistic than that![53]

This may be a good point to interject something most people may not think about. When I mention whole body healing throughout this writing, you know what I mean. The whole body has to heal to address chronic diseases. What you may miss in this thought is that everything in the body is connected. We as humans are one whole organism. If someone is diagnosed with a cardiovascular disease and they have severe inflammation in their blood vessels, the cause of the inflammation isn't just affecting the cardiovascular system, it's causing inflammation in the whole body; for example, in the intestines. Inflammation in these two areas can lead to numerous adverse health effects. I bring this up for a reason. You have probably noticed that one preventative measure can help in multiple areas of the body, because we are one whole organism. These examples have been given throughout this writing, and there are more to come. There are times when acute traumas happen to us and we need a certain area of the body treated, like a broken bone or even a reaction to an allergen like peanuts. But when it comes to something that requires whole body healing, like eczema, I feel that a holistic approach is far better. Something that conventional medicine is missing is this approach to healing because today, most conventional treatments are an acute treatment of symptoms that can have devastating side effects.

I will use my mother again as another example. Years ago, she was taking Maxalt as a prescribed medication to address migraine headaches. One of the side effects of this medication is a heart attack, and that's exactly what happened. By coincidence or God's grace, she was in an appointment with her doctor who was in the room with her when she had the attack. They realized it right away, gave her aspirin, and she was in the ER within minutes. She is fine today, and her heart is in great health, but what a scary situation. After this event, she still had migraine headaches, so what was she prescribed next? Well it's the drugs that are taking this country by storm and having devastating consequences.

OPIOIDS

She had been taking them for several years when migraines struck, but they don't treat what's causing the headache. They only cover up the pain, and cause addiction. She would get these narcotics from a pain clinic where they would be prescribed to her, and after years of taking these addicting drugs, she was starting to be abused by the staff. I will tell you this clinic was in Napa, California. They were accusing her of being a drug addict and trying to get these "medications" when she didn't need them. It infuriated me. That's the whole problem. These narcotics are prescribed for pain, and then people get addicted; as a result, they can't get the medication anymore, and then they turn to the streets to get the drugs that feed the addiction.

For the people at this clinic to accuse my mother of being a drug addict when they are the ones prescribing these drugs is crazy. I mentioned that Mom was using cannabis to wean herself off these drugs. She was also still a part of the pain clinic and received smaller doses of opioids to aid in coming off. Quitting cold turkey can have severe effects, including severe anxiety, body aches, difficulty sleeping, severe nausea, diarrhea, and vomiting. She made a mistake and mentioned she was using cannabis to ease any adverse effects that resulted from quitting. They told her if she tested positive for "drug use" that she would be kicked out of the clinic. This is double crazy! It's so ridiculous that it's both funny and infuriating at the same time. I don't know where you stand on marijuana, but to have it in the same category as these opioids or street drugs like heroine is ludicrous. To call it a Schedule 1 drug as the federal government does doesn't make sense. We will get into cannabis and the wonder that it is later in this book.

The fact that they would kick her out of a clinic where they got her addicted to these drugs in the first place, and at a time when she is taking it upon herself to get off them, is where the danger lies. I don't think this would have happened with my mom, but this situation is exactly one in which people are led to the streets to fill their addictions; and too many are ending up dead.

I can't imagine the number of other cases out there today that are not as lucky as my mother. I also can't believe that a medication is prescribed that would have such drastic side effects. It makes me wonder what is going on at the Food and Drug Administration (FDA). Can't they see that the medicine is right in the name of their organization. Food should be used as the Drugs that are to be Administered to patients. Not drugs that are synthesized to mimic these natural plant compounds.

Also concerning is what seemed to be a media push by The American Heart Association (AHA). Recently, they released a report warning that saturated fats like coconut oil and butter need to be reduced or replaced by "healthier" polyunsaturated, omega-6 fats like margarine and vegetable oils, such as corn, soybean, canola, and sunflower. They claim that these saturated oils raise LDL cholesterol levels and put you at risk of heart disease. We covered what is going on with these oils. What happened a few months later? The president of the AHA suffered a heart attack at a conference. My guess is that the he followed the recommendations that his association called for to reduce cardiovascular disease or coronary artery disease. Friends, the health advice from the AHA is the same as the advice from the FDA or the "myplate" recommendations. They are ass-backwards. Follow the two, and you are going to cause double the amount of inflammation in the body by eating fats that oxidize and rust you from the inside, or eight slices of bread a day which will do the same. Please be highly critical of health recommendations coming from government-run agencies.

Let's look at some more studies on the effects of coconut oil. Here is a 2003 animal study out of India: Beneficial effects of virgin coconut oil on lipid parameters and in vitro LDL oxidation. This study demonstrates the effects of virgin coconut oil in a wet extraction compared to a dry extraction. Total cholesterol was reduced as well as LDL, and HDL levels increased. Exactly opposite of what the AHA said would happen. [54]

Next, we have a study in an elderly group from 2015. A coconut extra virgin oil-rich diet increases HDL cholesterol and decreases waist circumference and body mass in coronary artery disease patients. 116 people who had coronary artery disease were broken into groups and given a diet with virgin coconut oil, and the others were given another diet. The results were a reduction in waist and neck circumference, and an increase in HDL. [55]

Here is a preliminary study from Spain involving patients with Alzheimer's dementia. Cognitive test scores improved in women who were given 40 milliliters of coconut oil per day. The medium chain triglycerides in coconut oil can supply energy to the brain and prevent neuron death, the cause of Alzheimer's. Diabetes was also a factor and the degree of the Alzheimer's in the patients affected the outcome. There is a lot more to study here, but what a great bode of the medicinal properties of coconut oil. [56]

I can't leave out a great technique of oral care when it comes to coconut oil, and that is oil pulling, or swishing coconut oil around in your mouth for 10-20 minutes. Please be aware not to swallow the oil and spit into the garbage, not down the drain. In probably the only study of its kind, 60 16-18-year-old boys and girls with gingivitis caused from plaque were monitored for 30 days. They added oil pulling to their oral hygiene routine and the outcome was reduced plaque formation, which in turn decreased the likelihood of gingivitis forming. [57]

INFLAMMATION

I point out inflammation for a purpose. There are a lot of topics that we have already covered that will address inflammation, but let's talk about it. Inflammation is usually the swelling in the lining of blood vessels, intestines, or joints. If the inflammation is chronic, diseases may form, like cancer, cardiovascular disease, neurological disorders, auto immune problems, arthritis, diabetes, and Alzheimer's.

What causes the inflammation to lead to these diseases? Smoking, drinking excess alcohol, SAD (standard American diet), free radicals, chemicals, GMOs, and stress. Some of these are unavoidable, and we are inundated with free radicals by walking down the street, especially people who live in big cities. Car, bus, and truck exhaust: we're inhaling it daily. Low levels of radiation from our cell phones, cell towers, airport body scanners, and X-rays at the dentist. I don't care what they say. It all adds up.

I find myself walking down the street and breathing in a very unhealthy way. I have lots of deep exhales if I pass a smoggy vehicle or an older model car that expels a lot of smoke when the light turns green. I essentially hold my breath until I feel it's a safer place to take in some decent quality air. Maybe I need to move out of the city?

So, what can we do to avoid all of this inflammation? Well, quitting smoking is an easy one, easily said at least. Reduce drinking, address stress, and avoid chemicals as much as you can. The biggest would be to change your diet and how you shop by avoiding genetically modified organisms (GMOs). We will cover this later.

Add in foods that have anti-inflammatory properties like flavonoids and resveratrol-rich foods. Dark unsweetened chocolate, dark berries, organic red wine, flaxseed (ground), pomegranate, pumpkin seeds, tart cherries, sesame seeds, blackberry, cranberry, garlic, grapes, and spices. We covered resveratrol as more of an anti-aging compound and touched on its cardiovascular protective properties, but here it is again as a great anti-inflammatory. Human trials with resveratrol are scarce, but here is some "first of its kind" science. In a 75-person long-term study from the American Journal of Cardiology, participants were given a resveratrol grape supplement and there were no side effects. Some of the participants were on statins, and the conclusion of the study was that resveratrol could compliment the standard of care when it comes to cardiovascular disease.[58]

I think everyone probably knows where I'm going in the spice category, but just in case you don't know, turmeric is a great anti-inflammatory. Turmeric is also a well-known spice in Indian cooking and contains a compound called curcumin. The list of benefits of curcumin is abundant, from reducing depression, to fighting oral plaque, to having therapeutic effects in pancreatic cancer.[59,60,61]

The most widely-known benefit is, of course, the anti-inflammatory properties. I personally don't need to research the benefits of curcumin because for me, it is an obvious form of medicine. But when I did, I found over 2,500 related articles on Pub Med, maybe even more. I found a lot of other uses for turmeric like the ones above, but most were inflammation-related issues. The one that stood out to me was a Cambridge study published in the *British Journal of Nutrition.* It concluded that a "natural occurring food substance with no known human toxicity" was a therapy that could be used to treat irritable bowel syndrome, a devastating condition that can lead to cancer. The same therapy could also be applied to many autoimmune issues, many of which are very prevalent in children with autism.[62]

You have to love those results! Food is medicine!

CANNABIS

This may be a surprise to some, and in this section, if you haven't already, please open your mind a bit. This is another example of the government taking your health into their hands. We covered inflammation, and another great anti-inflammatory plant is cannabis, or hemp. The various forms of CBD, THC, and THCa have tremendous anti-inflammatory properties, and can treat anxiety, affect cancer cells, and serve as a major medicine for those suffering from epilepsy or seizures.

Let's start here. The United States Health and Human Services (HHS) holds a patent on cannabis or marijuana, stating the cannabinoids can be useful in the treatment of neurodegenerative diseases such as Alzheimer's, Parkinson's, and dementia.[63] Science is also finding many other uses for this natural plant, like the treatment of cancer. The Drug Enforcement Agency (DEA) has marijuana or cannabis as a schedule I drug, along with heroin, LSD, ecstasy, methamphetamine (meth) and peyote. A Schedule I drug is classified as a substance or drug with no current medical use, and a high potential for abuse. It is also in a category as a hallucinogen.

We can see the contradiction here from government agencies. We also see the medical uses cannabis has with major degenerative disease; so why is the DEA continuing to treat cannabis as an addictive drug and not realizing that it's medicine? Who knows?

I will state that nobody has EVER overdosed or died when directly smoking or ingesting cannabis.

I imagine in the near future that this DEA ruling or law will change as it has been doing state-by-state. As of this writing, eight states have legalized cannabis for recreational use, and around 31 (including the eight) have approved medical marijuana. That's most of the states voting for cannabis as a drug with medicinal properties, and science is backing that up.

As a teenager, I probably did abuse marijuana, but I knew very few who didn't. Growing up in Napa, we were just south of the Emerald triangle, Humboldt, Mendocino, and Ukiah, where probably the best marijuana in the world is grown. We were as much connoisseurs of cannabis as were the people of fine wines that grow in the region. We all knew that the day would come when it would be legal, and about 24 years later, California has legalized it. Back then, I knew of friends' parents that were sick with cancer that were smoking marijuana to feel better after experiencing the side effects of the treatments that they were going through. We have come a long way since then, and it's too bad we didn't know what we know now about other forms of cannabis that are highly medicinal.

Now before you dismiss me as some hippie stoner in California, know that I don't smoke anymore. I know smoking helps a lot of people with adverse conditions, but if you are only using cannabis for recreational purposes, I think you are missing the point. When the good, fun feeling wasn't there anymore I stopped; I was probably 19 or 20 years old. It was easy, there was no addiction.

I do, however, use CBD almost daily which has no THC. THC is the cannabinoid compound that gives marijuana the psychoactive effect, or the high. CBD is not a drug; it can be used as an overall well-being oil, and or an anti-inflammatory among the other many conditions it can treat. CBD is 100% legal, can be shipped across state lines, and is safe for anyone to use, even pets. I also used medical cannabis legally, with a card, and applied some products that do contain low amounts of THC. These are a form of prevention for me, and that's exactly what I told the doctor when they prescribed my medical marijuana card.

I do not advise breaking any laws to be able to take cannabis for medical reasons, but there are many who are.

People are sick, and they are informed and educated on the benefits of cannabis. They have seen themselves get better when taking cannabis and seen themselves get worse when they didn't have access to it. I have listened to stories of people relocating their entire family to Colorado, so their young child could legally receive the medicine that stops severe seizures that happen up to a thousand times a day. Or a mother fighting pancreatic cancer in New York before they had medical dispensaries. She established a residency in California, so she could obtain her medicine. She did break the law and carried cannabis back with her to NYC, crossing over state lines.

Another heartbreaking story was a woman who had an inoperable brain tumor. The oncologists were pushing her to undergo high-dose, full-cranial radiation treatments. The woman had heard of cannabis. She was also from the east coast; she flew to Oregon to buy her medicine, and then flew back with it and broke the law. She finally gave into radiation but also kept up with the cannabis as well. Not too long after, she died. The autopsy showed that she had zero cancer in her brain but died of radiation-induced brain damage. A shocking, sad story that should never had happened. These stories and more were introduced to me after watching a series called the Sacred Plant, which was conceived by founder John Malanca and his wife Corinne. Corrinne's father was fighting cancer and went through the standard treatment to no avail. The doctors sent him home to die. While in hospice, John and Corinne discovered cannabis and the power it possesses. After giving it to their father, he got better and is still alive today. I highly recommend watching this series. It is the most informative information I have seen in one place at one time. If you want to know the truth behind cannabis, you owe it to yourself to watch.

I also mentioned my mother who is using cannabis to help wean herself off highly addictive opioids that were prescribed to her. My mother is using a non-addictive plant with numerous medicinal purposes, a Schedule I drug, to help her become non-addicted to all of the prescribed Schedule 2 drugs. She didn't take all these drugs, but they're all in the same category: Oxytocin, Vicodin, Dilaudid, Adderall, and Ritalin. These are all highly addictive prescriptions. Talk about ass-backward situations: a natural plant that grows in the wild is considered more dangerous than these toxic pharmaceuticals that are ravaging this nation's health.

It's a shame that people have to break the law to get the medicine that is going to help them win the fight against major diseases. Well-known celebrity neurosurgeon Sanjay Gupta of CNN completely reversed his opinion of cannabis and did a news special a few years back that involved stories like the ones above. If you want the true story of how cannabis became illegal, and much more knowledge of the science behind the medicinal properties again, watch and support the Sacred Plant.

Here is a fact that can be very beneficial – an epigenetic preventative measure you can take into your own life. Many cells, if not every cell in our body, contain cannabinoid receptors, or the endocannabinoid system. This system predominately lies in the nervous and immune systems. Cannabinoids are the compounds that make up cannabis. There are around 115 cannabinoids in a plant. Isn't it ironic that our body has systems in place to receive the compounds from a natural plant; really no surprise here. But who would interfere with this natural process? A government agency.

Here is a 2017 study out of Iran: Standardized *sativa* extract attenuates tau and stathmin gene expression in the melanoma cell line. This research looks at the gene expression of two proteins that are relevant in melanoma metastasis. They came to discover that the sativa strain of cannabis decreased gene expression, and in turn, metastatic melanoma. Cannabis affecting the epigenetics of cells fights and aids in curing deadly skin cancer. It's a nontoxic natural plant that can double as a preventative as well.[64]

Another 2006 study from Spain titled, Cannabinoid receptors as novel targets for the treatment of melanoma, states that the only effective measures against melanoma are prevention and early detection. There has been vast research in this area and the study concludes that cannabinoids inhibit the growth of melanoma cells, but do not affect normal cells. They find cannabis and cannabinoids to be chemotherapeutic.[65]

An article out of the *Journal of Investigative Dermatology* concludes that THC activates autophagy, and apoptosis in melanoma cells in vitro. Sativex, approved in the UK, was the botanical used to perform this research, and the study states this finding warrants clinical evaluation.[66]

This is eye-opening research and hopefully it would help a skeptic realize that marijuana is not an evil plant that turned Mexicans into killers or drove people mad in the 1930's like the propaganda film *Reefer Madness* led people to believe. Again, it's a plant and no one in the world has ever directly overdosed and died from the consumption or smoking of cannabis.

I witnessed the power of cannabis oil firsthand. I always knew that cannabis was a medicine, and I was introduced to a film called *Run from the Cure*. It was made by Rick Simpson, a Canadian who "cooked" cannabis oil and was healing people in the area he lived. The oil is a very thick tar-like resin and is very concentrated. Essentially, cannabis oil is made by leaching out the oils of the cannabis bud with a solvent, and then cooking the liquid down in a rice cooker that doesn't allow the oil to reach above 300 degrees Fahrenheit. The oil can be taken orally or used topically.

When I was in my 20's and probably until I was 30, I always had a blemish on the side of my nose. This is a gross example, but it would form a whitehead, then partially heal, but it never fully healed or went away; it was my "perma zit." Rick Simpson did an experiment on himself. He was diagnosed with skin cancer in multiple places. He had some cancer removed surgically and the other areas he treated with his cannabis oil. The locations where the oil was administered went way, healed, and never returned. The surgically removed cancer came back and he used the oil to heal that as well. After seeing this, I used cannabis oil on my perma zit, and it never came back after a few days of adding oil to a small band aid and leaving it on overnight! Thank you, Rick Simpson!

If you feel that cannabis may be a good choice for your health or if you want to use it to fight a disease, there are some precautions you should be aware of. Cannabis is not a "one size fits all" therapy. Dosing is different for everyone, especially if you are using medicine that does contain THC. People handle the "high" in very different ways. I would advise working with doctors who are experienced in the different strains of cannabinoids, and what ailments they work well with in treating. Also work with physicians who are experienced in the beginning stages of dosing.

Two doctors stood out to me and were interviewed on the Sacred Plant. The first was Dr. Dustin Sulak out of Falmouth, Maine. He has a great website, Healer.com. It is a great resource for anyone using cannabis in either beginning or advanced stages. Another would be Dr. Allan Frankel out of Santa Monica, California. Both of these doctors have had great success in treating people with cannabis.

Cannabinoids have anti-tumor activity.[67] I hope this has become clear, and hopefully if you were a cannabis skeptic, you may give it some consideration now. We covered inflammation, and here are two studies, from the Department of Epidemiology and Biostatistics, Michigan State University and Clinical Science, which examine the smoking of cannabis as an anti-inflammatory and also as an aid in an acutely inflamed colon.[68,69]

Would you think the seeds of hemp could be beneficial as well? You betcha! Hemp seeds are a great source of plant-based proteins, with about nine grams of protein per three tablespoons of seed. They are very easily digestible and are about 30% fat, which is high in omega-3 and omega-6 fatty acids. These fatty acids then give the seeds a cardioprotective benefit.[70] Also, THC may have cardioprotective features as well, as this 2010 study, "The cardiac and haemostatic effects of dietary hempseed", shows. Here, low doses were given to diabetic animals. The THC helped aid in cardio organ function, which reduced the diabetic effects of cardiovascular disease.[71]

The list of benefits goes on – cannabis has been shown to aid symptoms of epilepsy, childhood epilepsy, brain tumor-related epilepsy, and chronic seizures. A quick search produced 28 articles related to the matter, and around 290 other topics, each relating to different diseases that cannabis can help treat. One plant, 290 diseases. Why are the powers that be suppressing this medicine?

GMO "GOD MOVE OVER"

I don't remember where I first heard that phrase, so I credit everyone I have heard say it, maybe it was Jeffery Smith.

I want to touch on an issue that is a controversial topic, the Genetically Modified Organism (GMO). There are heated debates over it. Advocates of GMOs state they are safe foods, they are superior forms of agriculture, and these crops have the ability to feed the world with increased yields, in areas where people still don't have abundant access to food.

The flip side is organic growing practices create the same if not more of a yield than GM crops and are safer. There are claims that GM foods can cause allergies in children, and that they use chemicals that are cancer-causing. Contamination is also a grave concern. GM crops can contaminate non-GM crops with either their genes through fertilization, or the pesticides and herbicides that they are sprayed with. The contamination of soil with toxic chemicals is even reaching into rivers and streams, contaminating whole ecosystems.

You can probably guess where I stand on the issue. Overall, I'm not a fan of interfering with nature. Nature will always find a way to do what it was intended to do. One example is the use of these chemicals on crops. The crop is genetically modified to resist the chemical and kill the weeds, fungus, and insects that interfere with crop yield. This is now creating new species of super weeds that are resistant to the chemicals that were made to kill them, and in turn, more chemicals are needed to address the problem. This is a prime example of nature finding a way to survive what man is trying to alter. Not to mention, growing crops that have been modified to resist toxic chemicals? Organics also spray chemicals to some extent when other organic methods are not working, but this food is nowhere near the toxicity of GMO crop spray. By law, organic chemicals must come from a natural source whereas conventional or GMO crops are sprayed with synthesized products.

GMOs don't really fit into the topic of this book, which is using natural holistic treatments to fight and prevent disease, but avoiding GMOs as a preventative measure is essential to your health. It should be addressed, especially if you are not familiar with the topic. Let's look at what's out there on GMOs.

You may know that Monsanto is one of the biggest GMO producers in the world. They produce the chemical glyphosate, which is prevalent in the well-known weed killer Roundup. Roundup has been around for decades. I remember using it as a kid with my parents in the yard. If I only knew what I know now. Monsanto claims that Roundup is a safe chemical and has no adverse impact on humans. There is controversy that Monsanto has covered up the fact that it *is* toxic to humans. The fight in the United States persists today and also in Europe. This may be biased, but it seems Monsanto is trying to take over the world with their GM crops and chemicals. But Europe is not putting up with it. All 28 European nations have passed laws requiring GMOs to be labeled, and Ireland is the most recent EU country to ban the cultivation of GM crops. Period.[72,73]

In the U.S. and Canada, many are still fighting for GMO labeling as a basic human right – you should know what's in your food. Rachel Parent of Toronto, Canada is an activist who's been advocating for labeling and informing people about GMOs since she was a minor. She has been a TED Talk speaker and founded Kids Right to Know. If you want to get involved and make a change for the better, follow her and her work! Non-labeling is criminal in my book. People should be informed and able to choose what they are consuming, and one argument you will hear if you get involved in the controversy is:

If GMOs are so safe for humans,
then why the fight to label?

Being a resident of California, the land of fruits and nuts, I've been more susceptible to hearing news about this fight going on between Monsanto and everyone who opposes its products. It may also be safe to say that Californians may be more impacted by Roundup and glyphosate than most due to the heavy agriculture business in the state, and even its use in viticulture or wine making, and in parks or in private residential use. I know in the past I have driven down the road in Napa and gone right through clouds of chemical spray from a nearby vineyard. It's another instance where I have to roll up the window and hold my breath, though these chemicals can cause harm by coming into contact with your skin or eyes as well.

In April 2018, Monsanto headed to court in California to defend Roundup being labeled as a carcinogen in the state. This label would warn consumers that the products contain chemicals or ingredients that are cancer-causing. This came after studies from the World Health Organization showed glyphosate as a probable carcinogen. Under Proposition 65, where labeling is required of products that are known to cause cancer and other adverse reactions, California won the court battle.[74]

After this victory, it seemed to have spawned thousands of lawsuits against Monsanto from people who have developed non-Hodgkin's lymphoma. Some of these lawsuits are led by Robert F. Kennedy Jr. (RFK) of the nonprofit Children's Health Defense, formerly the World Mercury Project. RFK is an environmental lawyer; he fights for issues that no one wants to touch. Recently, he was a part of another lawsuit that showed the Department of Health and Human Services has not been conducting vaccine safety research as it is required by law – for three decades.[75] As of this writing, RFK is in San Francisco leading one of the first highly publicized cases of these lawsuits. Dewayne Johnson developed non-Hodgkin's lymphoma after exposure to glyphosate in the chemicals he used as a groundskeeper. The suit also claims that Monsanto hid evidence that showed glyphosate was a cancer-causing herbicide.[76]

Regardless of how these lawsuits turn out, I want to point out to you that Monsanto has now merged with parent company Bayer and the name Monsanto will go by the wayside. It's an obvious strategic move by these two chemical companies. But make no mistake, though you may not hear the name Monsanto anymore, these issues are still very much at hand.[77]

Update: Dewayne Johnson was awarded some 290 million dollars after a unanimous decisions of the Jury in the case against Monsanto. Very recently (October 20, 2018) the judge may overturn some of the award, which to some brings into questions the process of our judicial system.

What is other science telling us about GMOs and the fitted chemicals produced to treat the crops? Dr. Arnaldo Cantani, an Italian physician and non-GMO proponent said, "Genetic engineering poses innovative ethical and social concerns, as well as serious challenges to the environment, human health, animal welfare, and the future of agriculture."[78]

In a look at the health risks in children and the severe rise in food allergies, the above quote was the conclusion in a review of genetic manipulation of food. Another interesting study to add to the controversy is a comparison of three studies that Monsanto preformed on their own GM corn varieties. This comparison study looks at Bacillus thuringiensis (or Bt) toxin, an insecticide used on GM corn. Monsanto claims this protein that produces the toxin is only a danger to insects and is safe for humans and animals. Rats in a control group were fed GM corn and some not, they were tested at weeks 5 and 14. There were lots of factors that differentiate the groups and their outcomes like, sex, weeks of feeding, and the dosing, but the effects were found primarily in the liver and kidney. Also, the heart, adrenal glands, and spleen were taken into consideration, and the conclusion was that toxicity was present in these areas.[79]

As this is a disturbing study, and appears to expose manipulated science from Monsanto, one has to wonder if it is even possible or legal for companies to conduct research on their own products? If they find a negative outcome, are they going to shut down their moneymakers? Or spend the extra it will take to change formulation?

I'm going to take you back to the Truth about Cancer conference I attended. Here was the first time I was introduced to Jeffery Smith, a known opponent of GMOs and an expert in the field.

His film, *Genetic Roulette* and his book, *Seeds of Deception,* are content you should access if you are concerned about what you are reading right now. Also, his website has great GMO education at responsibletechnology.com. There are more science articles like the one above listed there.[80] Various studies are troubling and have very concerning outcomes, like Roundup causing placental cell death, GM crops threatening human fertility and health safety, and GM corn causing issues with immune systems in mice. He also touched on potential fraud and autism, and subjects like gluten disorders. This information is all very real and relevant, and the contamination of the planet is at stake here.

Dr. Patrick Gentempo is also another leader in the GMO space. He launched a series called GMOs Revealed. This is another great way to educate yourself on the dangers of GMOs and the havoc they are creating across the globe.

Another very controversial topic is autism. What is causing it? Are kids born this way? Is it genetic? Is there environmental exposure that could be causing it? Along with controversial topics, the people who speak about them are often caught in the crosshairs of one side or the other. Stephanie Seneff is a prime example of this. She's in the field of computer science at MIT and a researcher. Mrs. Seneff was one of the first, if not only, researchers to point out autism's exponential growth. The ratio of autism has gone from one in thousands to one in 25, and that ratio is increasing faster as time goes by.

Seneff has published many papers looking at glyphosate as a cause of many health issues that plague the U.S. and the world today. These problems include autism, food allergies, microbiome issues, and autoimmune issues. Here is a 2014 article from Interdisciplinary Toxicology that provides links between glyphosate and celiac disease, or to a lesser extent, gluten disorders.[81] The paper points directly toward Roundup and glyphosate as the cause of these epidemics by detoxifying pathways that are disrupted after coming in contact with glyphosate. In one of a series of articles entitled "Glyphosate, pathways to modern diseases III: manganese, neurological diseases, and associated pathologies," Seneff looks at neurological disorders, Alzheimer's, Parkinson's, and depression. Manganese is an essential metal for humans, animals, and plants. Glyphosate acts as a chelator against manganese, and it is secreted out of the body, which could aid in development of these ailments.[82]

To round this section out (no pun intended), I want to ask you a question. If you wanted to buy an apple and had two side-by-side, one being a natural apple that may have been treated with chemicals derived from natural compounds; the other with genes manipulated in a lab by a company to resist the chemicals that the same company created, which would you choose? I've heard some arguments that millions of meals have been consumed in the world that contained GM products, and there hasn't been an issue. Yes, I will agree if you eat a GM apple, you probably are not going to be rushed to the emergency room. Maybe not even if you eat one a day for a month. But think about the health of our nation at this moment. Where are we right now? We are a very sick nation, and it just so happens that our food is unlabeled. If you are uneducated and don't know what to look for, you are most likely eating GMOs. If you are buying a non-organic product and want to be sure it is GMO-free, look for a Non-GMO project verification symbol. If you don't see one, there is a good chance you are consuming GMOs.

GUT HEALTH AND MICROBIOME

Let's start with a history lesson from 19th century France.[83] There were two rival biologists, Antoine Bechamp and Louis Pasteur. You may see the name Pasteur and think that it sounds like the root of the word *pasteurization*, and you would be correct. Pasteurization occurs when you heat an item like milk to kill any germs that may be present. Pasteur's thinking was that germs cause disease, so if we kill them, less people will suffer from these diseases. Bechamp's theory was the opposite; germs were there to help balance diseased dysfunctional cells and were a byproduct of the disease. As you have probably figured out, Pasteur's theory won out, but it looks like Bechamp was actually right with all of the imbalances people are now experiencing in today's world. And to put it mildly, I haven't heard of anyone catching a disease from eating sauerkraut or kimchi.

In recent years, we have really discovered the importance of the microbiome. You may already be familiar with this term, and you would be correct if you said that it lies in your gut. But it is also much more than that. Your microbiome extends from your colon through your whole digestive tract, to your lungs and respiratory system, up to your mouth and nose, and into your brain, and it's all connected, like we know everything in our bodies is connected.

Here is a little fact I would like to interject. In the morning when you wake before your first bowel movement, you are made up of more microbial cells than human cells; that's right, essentially you are not human but a bug!

Everything affects your microbiome, like the food you eat. How was the food treated? Was the chicken you ate crammed in a cage in a stressful environment, or was it able to roam free? This is engrained into the microbiome of the animal, which can in turn have an effect on your own microbiome (e.g., the stress you feel). Great stress can lead to inflammation and an acidic environment in your body, leaving you open to all sorts of chronic conditions. Even the air quality you are exposed to can have an effect. Are you always indoors, in an office, in a high-rise with air-conditioning, then going home to stale house-air, or always on an airplane in recycled air? All of these things affect your microbiome very quickly. The difference between these situations and being outside in fresh air, gardening in your yard, is a difference that could affect your lifespan. Everything can affect the stability of your microbiome.

In the environments where the microbiome is adversely affected, it can in turn lead to a compromise in your immune system. I might be preaching to the choir here, but 80% of our immune system is in our gut, making up the vast majority of our microbiome and obviously our immune system. Think about that when you eat a meal that is of lesser quality or full of chemicals or additives. When you eat food, it doesn't only go to your stomach then get broken down through your intestine and then excreted on the other side, it literally affects your whole immune system. Do you want to fuel your immune system with burgers and fries or avocado and kale?

Dr. Zach Bush is a foremost expert in microbiome health. Again, in an interview with Naomi Whittle on her series The Real Skinny on Fat, Dr. Bush talks about this fact and also how it can take some work to change your diet for the better. Dr. Bush explains how the bacteria in our gut and our microbiome becomes accustomed to the foods we eat and in turn can cause you to crave those same foods. When you try to eat something healthier you may have a bad reaction, and the brain reinforces that these good foods are causing bad things to happen.

So, when I make a statement like do you want to feed your immune system burger and fries or avocado and kale, the answer looks easy. But when you take this into real life to make the real change, it can become much more challenging. It takes time to make the shift and there may be some adverse reactions along the way, but in time, you can retrain the bacteria in your gut to signal for these foods that will benefit your gut and overall health at the same time. It makes perfect sense, and Dr. Bush is such an amazing person to listen to about this most important part of our health.

Gut health is crucial! There is a constant "competition" happening in our intestines. A fine balance needs to be created between good and bad bacteria, or the microbes that call the gut home; we need both. When it's one or the other, we may fall into dysbiosis, a large imbalance which usually leaves us with less good bacteria. This can lead to weakening of the immune system or even tricking it into attacking our own bodies' normal functions or cells; in other words, it spurs autoimmune diseases.

Dysbiosis can occur in many ways, but one major way is through what's used when the body is already sick. The culprit that really has an effect on the microbiome is prescribed antibiotic medications. Kind of like giving chemo to an already sick cancer patient, the chemo kills all cells good and bad. Antibiotics, like chemo, will kill all good and bad bacteria in the gut. This may help kill the infection that is making you sick, but at the same time, it leaves your immune system stripped of everything, leaving you open to more sickness or disease. Also, as you are prescribed more and more, you can become resistant to these antibiotics, which can become a vicious cycle. I know of a lot of people who will go to the doctor in hope of being prescribed an antibiotic for a minor illness, and they sometimes get them.

I once had a urinary tract infection, went to get it checked out, and was given an antibiotic. I filled the prescription but didn't take it until I tried to heal the infection naturally using grapefruit essential oil internally. I also used cannabis oil, rubbing it into certain palaces, and the infection went away in a few days. Whether we can credit the holistic approach or if the infection took its course, who knows? Either way I was happy I didn't have to use the antibiotic and have to do extra work to rebuild the bacteria ratio in my gut, which could have left me open to another illness.

I also once had strep throat; this was undiagnosed. I didn't go to the doctor, but I know what strep feels and looks like. My throat was on fire and the white blotches were unmistakable. Again, I used a holistic approach, by supporting my immune system with very high doses of vitamin C, B-17 pills, and zinc, and also by gargling a mixture of apple cider vinegar, Himalayan pink salt, a little water, oregano, and peppermint essential oil. I gargled this 15-20 times per day. The peppermint created some temporary relief while the other ingredients did the work to kill the strep. As I have in the past with strep, I could have gone to an urgent care facility or the doctor, who surely would have prescribed an antibiotic, but I decided to treat it holistically. In about three days, I was back to normal. Again, whether the strep took its course or my treatment killed it, we won't know, but I do know I kept my gut healthier and didn't compromise my immune system by taking an antibiotic.

Now it's not only about antibiotics that are prescribed. There is another source of microbiome disturbance that's being administered through conventionally farmed wildlife. I mentioned this earlier with farm-raised fish, but when all of these animals are jammed together to be raised for meat consumption, their habitat needs to be treated to avoid disease spreading rampantly through the herd. These antibiotics are in the meat and absorbed by our microbiome, adding to the problems we're addressing.

A meta-analysis of over 4,000 papers looked at antibiotics used to treat urinary tract infections and respiratory infections. Several studies looked at the outcome of antibiotic resistance and found that this can create organisms that adapt to and become resistant to the antibiotics, and can even start to become resistant to second-line antibiotic use.[84]

Some issues that can arise and alert you to a malnourished gut can be respiratory issues, skin issues like acne, and reproductive or urinary issues. That is the start of the downward spiral. It starts with a compromised gut, then becomes an infection, then leads to further compromising the gut with antibiotic use, and then the gut becomes resistant to these medications.

We also have to realize the other toxicities we are treating our food with that are taking a toll on our guts. This even applies to the process to repair them. Pesticides and herbicides in GMO foods are all causing major toxicity that can hinder a repair process or create these issues in the first place.

Keep an eye on the "dirty dozen," a list you can find on multiple websites which informs you of conventionally grown foods that are known to have a high amount of chemicals used in their growth, and can also have a high amount of residual toxic residue. Always try to buy these organic or avoid them all together if that is not an option. Even washing these fruits and vegetables is not enough; these foods have been modified to resist the chemicals and well, you know the rest. But to back it up, here is a study that looks at glyphosate and the harm it can cause on the friendly bacteria in our gut.[85] "A reduction of beneficial bacteria in the gastrointestinal tract by ingestion of glyphosate could disturb normal gut bacteria."

Our gut is sometimes called our second brain, but something you may not know is that our gut actually controls our brain. It is our first brain and sends much more information to our actual brain than the brain sends to the gut. This makes perfect sense if you look at a known irritant like wheat. Wheat is everywhere, it's almost unavoidable, and what people with wheat sensitivities know is that it's very difficult for humans to break down. People without wheat sensitivities should know this fact as well. Even if you don't feel the immediate effect of wheat, know that it is most likely causing damage to your gut and health. There are aver 200 science-recognized diseases that have been researched with the link to wheat. Let's name some big ones: celiac disease, autoimmune diseases, schizophrenia, diabetes, psoriasis, and irritable bowel syndrome (IBS). Some that may be less known are: Down syndrome, autism spectrum disorders, osteoporosis, epilepsy, liver disease, migraine disorders, food allergies, and dysbiosis.

How could one food product cause all of these ailments? Inflammation. Our bodies can't break down the gluten in wheat, and this causes an irritation to our immune system, and this invader triggers an attack. Think of our gut lining as a porous cheesecloth-lined sausage casing. When we digest food, it is simulated in the gut and the nutrients get through the porous gut lining and into the bloodstream. Then it is delivered to our cells. Irritants like wheat trigger an immune response and inflammation because they can't be broken down. This constant inflammation then leads to intestinal permeability or leaky gut. The pores of the intestinal lining become enlarged which leads not only to irritants leaking through but possibly anything that is digested. Your body now views anything, even good foods, as an invader and this is how autoimmune issues are developed. Your body has the potential to create antibodies to almost everything you eat.

Okay, so now we have a leaky gut — what do we do about it? Literally last night, September 27, 2018, I was introduced to a product that Dr. Zach Bush and team have created called Restore. It's essentially a sterilized water that has been suspended with ancient soil. This soil contains vast amounts of microbial benefits for your microbiome. It's much more scientific than that explanation but you can take a deeper look at the science by reading Dr. Bush's whitepaper, Redox Molecule Protection of Tight Junctions NIH Grant Application 1R43DK103422-01. [86] This supplement has the ability to reverse leaky gut that has been caused by toxins, chemicals (glyphosate), or foods like gluten. What a great relief this could bring to so many people who are suffering from these microbiome issues, and also what a way to fight and prevent all these ailments that come with poor gut health. Check out https://shop.restore4life.com

Another expert in the field of gut health is Dr. Robert Scott Bell. Like many of the experts I've encountered, I was introduced to Dr. Bell at The Truth about Cancer, and he also has a daily radio show. His protocol to heal the microbiome is a wonder called colloidal silver. I had heard about silver as a holistic "medicine," but Dr. Bell drove home the benefits of silver. If you do a Google search, you'll probably see a picture of someone who looks like a blue Santa Claus. There was a man who did turn blue, a possible side effect of taking low-quality silver or homemade silver where the particles are not broken down into nanoparticles. A proper silver to use would be one made by Sovereign Silver — Bioactive Silver

Hydrosol. This silver is also a liquid with the nanoparticles suspended in it. They are so small that the liquid is clear, and that's the benefit. Smaller particles cover more surface area and can be quickly processed out of the body after they do their work. Silver can be used as immune support and has many other purposes. When Dr. Bell spoke, he told a story about his mother. She had eaten something bad and had food poisoning coming on. He directed her to drink a bottle of silver. Now neither of us would normally suggest doing something like this but it was the right time and place to "put a fire out", as he put it. By the way, I didn't see her in the audience but I'm pretty sure she wasn't blue.

Silver works by binding to DNA in cells aiding in the respiration of the cells and helping it to create energy as well as remove waste products. It can be used for colds, first aid, like burns or bug bites, and to help heal scar tissue. It also relieves eczema when applied topically and aids in healing the gut. Plus, it is antiviral and antimicrobial.

When using silver, it is a direct therapy, meaning the silver needs to be applied directly to the source, like a cut or wound, or in the case of food poisoning, directly to the stomach. Another great supplement to take for gut health is aloe vera juice. This is where we are able to deliver the silver directly to the gut. Aloe juice is not absorbed by the stomach. It goes straight through to the gut, so mixing the silver with aloe and drinking it will provide a direct application. The silver will heal tissue problems like permeability, help remove viruses, fungus, bad bacteria, and even parasites, and it will communicate with the microbiome.

I mentioned that I was a chef, and I have burned myself more times than I care to remember. Now when I burn myself, the first thing I do is go for the silver. I know burns. I know how they feel, how bad they are, whether they will blister. I'm kind of a burn expert. After using silver, I can tell you it provides instant relief; there is no pain or burning feeling, almost instantly. Burns that I know would have blistered do not and they usually heal a few days faster than normal; it truly is amazing stuff. Sovereign Silver also makes a gel that is a first aid treatment that I use on burns, or any other skin irritation. I highly recommend the stuff! And if you still don't believe me, here is some science to back it up.[87] From a 2009 article in Biotechnology Advances, silver nanoparticles are being accepted as an antimicrobial and antibiotic resistance tool, and the nanoparticle technology is being picked up by various medical applications, like dressings, devices, gels, and lotions. It's yet another naturally occurring substance being used to treat what pharma medicine can't.

WHAT'S THIS BOOK ABOUT AGAIN?

opefully you laughed at that title, because hopefully you have learned some deep knowledge that has struck a chord for you, maybe even given you an Aha! moment. I truly hope so. I hope you have found at least one tidbit of new information that could lead you down a path of prevention and healing. Like I mentioned before, I'm no expert. I'm a professional chef with some street cred as a health coach, but I felt the need to write this book. I felt the need to share what I have learned. This info is out there, and it's easy to find, but it's finding the first bit that takes you down the rabbit hole. I feel blessed and lucky to have stumbled upon such a path of knowledge, and I love the feeling of being able to take care of myself. If I had a family, I would be taking care of them as well, so maybe that's it. Maybe if you have read this, you are now family. I have shared enough personal stories about myself and mom.

I also feel like I'm a part of a family. The Truth about Cancer crew is family and anyone on the path of looking for the truth to keep yourself healthy is a part of this family as well. We need each other because sometimes it's not easy. There are a lot of naysayers out there, and there will continue to be as long as this symptom management healthcare system is what people look to for healing.

It was difficult to try and find the right order to place each topic, when everything is as connected as it is in our bodies. It feels as though it all needs to be communicated at once to achieve whole-body healing. Cancer felt like the best opener – it's such a devastating disease and also seems to be misunderstood. If there were no such thing as surgery, radiation, and chemo, I hope you'd still have some guidance to be able to heal. How do you feel about that? Would you know what to do? Would you know where to look? I hope there are tools you can use here to help in the fight.

I urge you to start researching the key points that may equip you if you ever need to fight a disease and also lead yourself toward greater prevention of disease in your life. Look into the plugs and name dropping. Look past the negative articles in your research and find the deeper truths for yourself. Be aware that it is absolutely true that companies ghostwrite articles that are full of Astroturf to confuse and make you doubt the truth only because it's a threat to their bottom line.

Start addressing the stress in your life, and look at your diet. Eating alkalizing foods is not going to have any adverse effects. Think about how that food can change how your genes act and recognize that you have the power of epigenetics on your side. Remember that there are two coaches you have in your corner, me and Chris Wark. By the way, I preordered his new book, *Chris Beat Cancer*, another tool.

Remember, specific treatments and natural compounds have a great effect on your health and can help you rid toxic products from your life. Essential oils are huge and hopefully you love resveratrol like I do. Remember, these same natural compounds can be used to help aid in a fight where conventional treatments are chosen. Essential oils and medicinal mushrooms help aid the process of chemo. Or take the free route to support yourself and just not eat: fasting. What a great tool toward prevention. Don't forget the others as well: achieve autophagy, and follow a ketogenic diet. Remember our contrarian Professor, Thomas Seyfried. Again, use these tools to fight and prevent the two biggest killers in the world today, cardiovascular disease and cancer.

Don't get caught in the confusion of government recommendations when it comes to your health. I hate to say it but the FDA is in bed with the CDC, and the AHA is recommending foods that 100% cause the conditions they exist to prevent. Follow the money and see that all of these agencies are influenced by "big" everything: pharma, agriculture, dairy, meat. Just remember the state of our health in this nation and the world. The DEA has categorized a natural plant the same as synthesized drugs that have no medicinal value and are highly addictive, while the same United States government holds patents on that very plant, as a medicine against neuro-degenerative diseases. One of the biggest chemical companies in the world essentially became a monopoly, and they want to grow food for the whole world, using their chemicals on our food, while stating it is all safe and wonderful in their own science.

The next time you go to the bathroom, remember that you are more bacteria than you are human.

All disease begins in the gut.
Illnesses do not come upon us out of the blue. They are developed from small daily sins against Nature. When enough sins have accumulated, illnesses will suddenly appear.
Let food be thy medicine and medicine be thy food.
— Hippocrates

REFERENCE NOTES

Introduction

1 Adams KM, Lindell KC, Kohlmeier M, Zeisel SH. Status of nutrition education in medical schools. Am J Clin Nutr. 2006;83(4):941S-944S. doi:10.1093/ajcn/83.4.941S

2 Gerson C. You cannot heal selectively. YouTube. https://www.youtube.com/watch?v=Zg4eYHo49Ul Published April 13, 2015. Accessed August 22, 2018.

3 Alsheikh-ali AA, Maddukuri PV, Han H, et al. Effect of the magnitude of lipid lowering on risk of elevated liver enzymes, rhabdomyolysis, and cancer: insights from large randomized statin trials. J Am Coll Cardiol. 2007;50(5):409-18. doi:10.1016/j.jacc.2007.02.073

4 Kim MJ, Nam ES, Paik SI. [The effects of aromatherapy on pain, depression, and life satisfaction of arthritis patients]. Taehan Kanho Hakhoe Chi.

5 2005;35(1):186-94. Korean. https://www.ncbi.nlm.nih.gov/pubmed/15778570 Accessed August 22, 2018.

6 Li B, Lv J, Wang W, Zhang D. Dietary magnesium and calcium intake and risk of depression in the general population: A meta-analysis. Aust N Z J Psychiatry. 2017;51(3):219-229. doi: 10.1177/0004867416676895

7 Al-karawi D, Al mamoori DA, Tayyar Y. The role of curcumin administration in patients with major depressive disorder: mini

meta-analysis of clinical trials. Phytother Res. 2016;30(2):175-83. doi: 10.1002/ptr.5524

8   Marx W, Kelly J, Marshall S, et al. The effect of polyphenol-rich interventions on cardiovascular risk factors in haemodialysis: A systematic review and meta-analysis. Nutrients. 2017;9(12) doi: 10.3390/nu9121345

9   Get the Facts. Campaign for safe cosmetics: a project of Breast Cancer Prevention Partners. http://www.safecosmetics.org/get-the-facts/ Accessed August 22, 2018.

10 Ji S. Research reveals how sugar causes cancer. GreenMedInfo. December 4, 2017. http://www.greenmedinfo.com/blog/research-reveals-how-sugar-causes-cancer Accessed August 22, 2018

11 Darbre PD, Aljarrah A, Miller WR, et al. Concentrations of parabens in human breast tumours. J Appl Toxicol. 2004;24(1):5-13. doi:10.1002/jat.958

12 Gerstein J. Your perfect shade is … "retinyl palmitate red"? Are the undisclosed ingredients in lipstick bad for you? Harper's Bazaar. March 28, 2018. www.harpersbazaar.com/beauty/makeup/advice/a485/lipstick-ingredients-020410   Accessed August 22, 2018.

Don't Wait Until You're Sick

1   Friberg S, Mattson S. On the growth rates of human malignant tumors: implications for medical decision making. J Surg Oncol. 1997 Aug;65(4):284-97 https://pdfs.semanticscholar.org/e5c8/b3dc69be1f60f5f5917bc4aa83ee5a1ac3d5.pdf Accessed August 22, 2018.

2   Jones H. Cancer cures more deadly than disease. Rethinking Cancer. Foundation for Advancement in Cancer Therapy: Non-Toxic Biological Approaches to the Theories, Treatments and Prevention of Cancer http://www.rethinkingcancer.org/resources/magazine-articles/2_1-2/

cancer-cures-more-deadly-than-disease.php Accessed August 22, 2018.

3   Morgan G, Ward R, Barton M. The contribution of cytotoxic chemotherapy to 5-year survival in adult malignancies. Clin Oncol (R Coll Radiol). 2004;16(8):549-60. https://www.ncbi.nlm. nih.gov/pubmed/15630849

4   Majalca B. Healing My Cancer. "Dr Bernardo's Lecture on the Importance of an Alkaline Diet." YouTube. Published September 6, 2013. https://www.youtube.com/watch?v=nsGTCy0oWPY Accessed August 22, 2018.

5   Schwalfenberg GK. The alkaline diet: is there evidence that an alkaline pH diet benefits health? J Environ Public Health. 2012;2012:727630. doi:10.1155/2012/727630

6   Brewer AK. The high pH therapy for cancer tests on mice and humans. Pharmacol Biochem Behav, 1984;21 Suppl 1:1-5. https:// s20975.pcdn.co/wp-content/uploads/2014/02/The-high-pH-therapy-for-cancer-tests-on-mice-and-humans.pdf Accessed August 22, 2018.

7   Tsuda H, Sata M, Kumabe T, et al. The preventive effect of antineoplaston AS2-1 on HCC recurrence. Oncol Rep. 2003;10(2):391-7. https://www.ncbi.nlm.nih.gov/pu bmed/?term=The+preventive+effect+of+antineoplaston +AS2-1+on+HCC+recurrence

8   Sugita Y, Tsuda H, Maruiwa H, et al. The effect of antineoplaston, a new antitumor agent on malignant brain tumors. Kurume Med J. 1995;42(3):133-40. https://www.ncbi.nlm.nih.gov/ pubmed/7474850

9   Burzynski SR, Janicki TJ, Weaver RA, et al. Targeted therapy with antineoplastons A10 and AS2-1 of high-grade, recurrent, and progressive brainstem glioma. Integr Cancer Ther. 2006;5(1):40-7. doi:10.1177/1534735405285380

10 Fujii, T., Yokoyama, G., Takahashi, H., et al. Preclinical studies of molecular-targeting diagnostic and therapeutic strategies against

breast cancer. Breast Cancer. 2008;15(1):73-8 doi:10.1007/s12282-007-0015-y.

11 De sanjosé S, Léoné M, Bérez V, et al. Prevalence of BRCA1 and BRCA2 germline mutations in young breast cancer patients: a population-based study. Int J Cancer. 2003;106(4):588-93. doi:10.1002/ijc.11271.

12 Breastcancer.org. Genetic test results: what to do if you've tested positive. http://www.breastcancer.org/symptoms/testing/genetic/pos_results Published February 19, 2018. Accessed August 23, 2018.

13 Veronesi A, De giacomi C, Magri MD, et al. Familial breast cancer: characteristics and outcome of BRCA 1-2 positive and negative cases. BMC Cancer. 2005;5:70. doi:10.1186/1471-2407-5-70.

14 Budroni M, Cesaraccio R, Coviello V, et al. Role of BRCA2 mutation status on overall survival among breast cancer patients from Sardinia. BMC Cancer. 2009;9:62. doi:10.1186/1471-2407-9-62.

15 Levin B, Lech D, Friedenson B. Evidence that BRCA1- or BRCA2-associated cancers are not inevitable. Mol Med. 2012;18:1327-37. doi: 10.2119/molmed.2012.00280

16 Hew KM, Walker AI, Kohli A, et al. Childhood exposure to ambient polycyclic aromatic hydrocarbons is linked to epigenetic modifications and impaired systemic immunity in T cells. Clin Exp Allergy. 2015;45(1):238-48. doi:10.1111/cea.12377.

17 Promkan M, Dakeng S, Chakrabarty S, et al. The effectiveness of cucurbitacin B in BRCA1_defective breast cancer cells. PLoS ONE. 2013;8(2):e55732. doi:10.1371/journal.pone.0055732.

18 Kowalska E, Narod SA, Huzarski T, et al. Increased rates of chromosome breakage in BRCA1 carriers are normalized by oral selenium supplementation. Cancer Epidemiol Biomarkers Prev. 2005;14(5):1302-6. doi:10.1158/1055-9965.EPI-03-0448.

19 Holcombe RF, Martinez M, Planutis K, et al. Effects of a grape-supplemented diet on proliferation and Wnt signaling in the colonic mucosa are greatest for those over age 50 and with

high arginine consumption. Nutr J. 2015;14:62. doi:10.1186/s12937-015-0050-z.

20 Brown VA, Patel KR, Viskaduraki M, et al. Repeat dose study of the cancer chemopreventive agent resveratrol in healthy volunteers: safety, pharmacokinetics, and effect on the insulin-like growth factor axis. Cancer Res. 2010;70(22):9003-11. doi:10.1158/0008-5472.CAN-10-2364.

21 Csiszar A, Labinskyy N, Podlutsky A, et al. Vasoprotective effects of resveratrol and SIRT1: attenuation of cigarette smoke-induced oxidative stress and proinflammatory phenotypic alterations. Am J Physiol Heart Circ Physiol. 2008;294(6):H2721-35. doi:10.1152/ajpheart.00235.2008

22 Ni X, Suhail MM, Yang Q, et al. Frankincense essential oil prepared from hydrodistillation of Boswellia sacra gum resins induces human pancreatic cancer cell death in cultures and in a xenograft murine model. BMC Complement Altern Med. 2012;12:253. doi:10.1186/1472-6882-12-253.

23 Ren P, Ren X, Cheng L, et al. Frankincense, pine needle and geranium essential oils suppress tumor progression through the regulation of the AMPK/mTOR pathway in breast cancer. Oncol Rep. 2018;39(1):129-137. doi:10.3892/or.2017.6067.

24 Beghelli D, Isani G, Roncada P, et al. Antioxidant and Immune System Regulatory Properties of Extracts. Oxid Med Cell Longev. 2017;2017:7468064. doi:10.1155/2017/7468064.

25 Khan MA, Ali R, Parveen R, et al. Pharmacological evidences for cytotoxic and antitumor properties of boswellic acids from Boswellia serrata. J Ethnopharmacol. 2016;191:315-323. doi:10.1016/j.jep.2016.06.053.

26 Gerbeth K, Meins J, Kirste S, et al. Determination of major boswellic acids in plasma by high-pressure liquid chromatography/mass spectrometry. J Pharm Biomed Anal. 2011;56(5):998-1005. doi:10.1016/j.jpba.2011.07.026.

27 Tayarani-najaran Z, Talasaz-firoozi E, Nasiri R, et al. Antiemetic activity of volatile oil from Mentha spicata and Mentha ×

piperita in chemotherapy-induced nausea and vomiting. Ecancermedicalscience. 2013;7:290. doi:10.3332/ecancer.2013.290

28 Kim YR. Immunomodulatory activity of the water extract from medicinal mushroom Inonotus obliquus. Mycobiology. 2005;33(3):158-62. doi:10.4489/MYCO.2005.33.3.158.

29 Paschall AV, Liu K. Epigenetic regulation of apoptosis and cell cycle regulatory genes in human colon carcinoma cells. Genom Data. 2015;5:189-191. doi:10.1016/j.gdata.2015.05.043.

30 Twardowski P, Kanaya N, Frankel P, et al. A phase I trial of mushroom powder in patients with biochemically recurrent prostate cancer: Roles of cytokines and myeloid-derived suppressor cells for Agaricus bisporus-induced prostate-specific antigen responses. Cancer. 2015;121(17):2942-50. doi:10.1002/cncr.29421.

31 Dorff TB, Groshen S, Garcia A, et al. Safety and feasibility of fasting in combination with platinum-based chemotherapy. BMC Cancer. 2016;16:360. doi:10.1186/s12885-016-2370-6.

32 Di biase S, Shim HS, Kim KH, et al. Fasting regulates EGR1 and protects from glucose- and dexamethasone-dependent sensitization to chemotherapy. PLoS Biol. 2017;15(3):e2001951. doi:10.1371/journal.pbio.2001951.

33 Longo V. What is the fasting mimicking diet? Prolon. https://prolonfmd.com/fasting-mimicking-diet/. Accessed August 23, 2018.

34 Brandhorst S, Choi IY, Wei M, et al. A periodic diet that mimics fasting promotes multi-system regeneration, enhanced cognitive performance, and healthspan. Cell Metab. 2015;22(1):86-99. doi:10.1016/j.cmet.2015.05.012.

35 Brown AJ. Low-carb diets, fasting and euphoria: is there a link between ketosis and gamma-hydroxybutyrate (GHB)? Med Hypotheses. 2007;68(2):268-71. doi:10.1016/j.mehy.2006.07.043.

36 Morselli E, Maiuri MC, Markaki M, et al. Caloric restriction and resveratrol promote longevity through the Sirtuin-1-dependent

induction of autophagy. Cell Death Dis. 2010;1:e10. doi: 10.1038/cddis.2009.8.

37 Siri-tarino PW, Sun Q, Hu FB, et al. Meta-analysis of prospective cohort studies evaluating the association of saturated fat with cardiovascular disease. Am J Clin Nutr. 2010;91(3):535-46. doi:10.3945/ajcn.2009.27725.

38 Cai B, Zhu Y, Ma Yi, et al. Effect of supplementing a high-fat, low-carbohydrate enteral formula in COPD patients. Nutrition. 2003;19(3):229-32. https://www.ncbi.nlm.nih.gov/pubmed/12620524

39 Hanahan D, Weinberg RA. Hallmarks of cancer: the next generation. Cell. 2011;144(5):646-74. doi: 10.1016/j.cell.2011.02.013.

40 Seyfried TN. Cancer as a mitochondrial metabolic disease. Front Cell Dev Biol. 2015;3:43. doi: 10.3389/fcell.2015.00043.

41 Warburg Hypothesis. Wikipedia. Edited June 23, 2018. https://en.wikipedia.org/w/index.php?title=Warburg_hypothesis&oldid=847194183

42 Seyfried TN, Flores RE, Poff AM, et al. Cancer as a metabolic disease: implications for novel therapeutics. Carcinogenesis. 2014;35(3):515-27. doi: 10.1093/carcin/bgt480.

43 Nebeling LC, Miraldi F, Shurin SB, et al. Effects of a ketogenic diet on tumor metabolism and nutritional status in pediatric oncology patients: two case reports. J Am Coll Nutr. 1995;14(2):202-8. https://www.ncbi.nlm.nih.gov/pubmed/7790697

44 Seyfried TN, Yu G, Maroon JC, et al. Press-pulse: a novel therapeutic strategy for the metabolic management of cancer. Nutr Metab (Lond). 2017;14:19. doi: 10.1186/s12986-017-0178-2.

45 İyikesici MS, Slocum AK, Slocum A, et al. Efficacy of metabolically supported chemotherapy combined with ketogenic diet, hyperthermia, and hyperbaric oxygen therapy for stage IV triple-negative breast cancer. Cureus. 2017;9(7):e1445. doi: 10.7759/cureus.1445.

46 Hemingway C, Freeman JM, Pillas DJ, Pyzik PL. The ketogenic diet: a 3- to 6-year follow-up of 150 children enrolled prospectively. Pediatrics. 2001;108(4):898-905. https://www.ncbi.nlm.nih.gov/pubmed/11581442

47 Kayyali HR, Luniova A, Abdelmoity A. Ketogenic diet decreases emergency room visits and hospitalizations related to epilepsy. Epilepsy Res Treat. 2016;2016:5873208. doi:10.1155/2016/5873208.

48 Al-zaid NS, Dashti HM, Mathew TC, et al. Low carbohydrate ketogenic diet enhances cardiac tolerance to global ischaemia. Acta Cardiol. 2007;62(4):381-9. doi:10.2143/AC.62.4.2022282.

49 Golomb BA. Implications of statin adverse effects in the elderly. Expert Opin Drug Saf. 2005;4(3):389-97. doi:10.1517/14740338.4.3.389.

50 Moosmann B, Behl C. Selenoprotein synthesis and side-effects of statins. Lancet. 2004;363(9412):892-4. doi:10.1016/S0140-6736(04)15739-5.

51 Aspirin for primary prevention of cardiovascular disease? Evid Based Med. 2010;15:31-33. doi:10.1136/ebm.15.1.31.

52 Dobnig H, Pilz S, Scharnagl H, et al. Independent association of low serum 25-hydroxyvitamin d and 1,25-dihydroxyvitamin d levels with all-cause and cardiovascular mortality. Arch Intern Med. 2008;168(12):1340-9. doi: 10.1001/archinte.168.12.1340.

53 Pareja-galeano H, Garatachea N, Lucia A. Exercise as a polypill for chronic diseases. Prog Mol Biol Transl Sci. 2015;135:497-526. doi: 10.1016/bs.pmbts.2015.07.019.

54 Nevin KG, Rajamohan T. Beneficial effects of virgin coconut oil on lipid parameters and in vitro LDL oxidation. Clin Biochem. 2004;37(9):830-5. doi:10.1016/j.clinbiochem.2004.04.010.

55 Cardoso DA, Moreira AS, De oliveira GM, et al. A coconut extra virgin oil-rich diet increases HDL cholesterol and decreases waist circumference and body mass in coronary artery disease patients. Nutr Hosp. 2015;32(5):2144-52. doi: 10.3305/nh.2015.32.5.9642.

56 Hu yang I, De la rubia ortí JE, Selvi sabater P, et al. [Coconut oil: non-alternative drug treatment against Alzheimer's disease]. Nutr Hosp. 2015;32(6):2822-7. doi:10.3305/nh.2015.32.6.9707. Spanish.

57 Peedikayil FC, Sreenivasan P, Narayanan A. Effect of coconut oil in plaque related gingivitis: a preliminary report. Niger Med J. 2015;56(2):143-7. doi: 10.4103/0300-1652.153406.

58 Tomé-carneiro J, Gonzálvez M, Larrosa M, et al. One-year consumption of a grape nutraceutical containing resveratrol improves the inflammatory and fibrinolytic status of patients in primary prevention of cardiovascular disease. Am J Cardiol. 2012;110(3):356-63. doi: 10.1016/j.amjcard.2012.03.030.

59 Al-karawi D, Al mamoori DA, Tayyar Y. The role of curcumin administration in patients with major depressive disorder: mini meta-analysis of clinical trials. Phytother Res. 2016;30(2):175-83. doi: 10.1002/ptr.5524.

60 Leite DP, Paolillo FR, Parmesano TN, et al. Effects of photodynamic therapy with blue light and curcumin as mouth rinse for oral disinfection: a randomized controlled trial. Photomed Laser Surg. 2014;32(11):627-32. doi: 10.1089/pho.2014.3805.

61 Dhillon N, Aggarwal BB, Newman RA, et al. Phase II trial of curcumin in patients with advanced pancreatic cancer. Clin Cancer Res. 2008;14(14):4491-9. doi: 10.1158/1078-0432. CCR-08-0024.

62 Epstein J, Docena G, Macdonald TT, et al. Curcumin suppresses p38 mitogen-activated protein kinase activation, reduces IL-1beta and matrix metalloproteinase-3 and enhances IL-10 in the mucosa of children and adults with inflammatory bowel disease. Br J Nutr. 2010;103(6):824-32. doi: 10.1017/S0007114509992510

63 United States Health and Human Services. Cannabinoids as antioxidants and neuroprotectants. Patent 6,630,507. October 7, 2003. http://patft.uspto.gov/netacgi/nph-Parser?Sect1= PTO1&Sect2=HITOFF&d=PALL&p=1&u=%2Fnetahtml%

2FPTO%2Fsrchnum.htm&r=1&f=G&l=50&s1=6630507.
PN.&OS=PN/6630507&RS=PN/6630507

64 Vaseghi G, Taki MJ, Javanmard SH. Standardized *sativa* extract attenuates tau and stathmin gene expression in the melanoma cell line. Iran J Basic Med Sci. 2017;20(10):1178-1181. doi: 10.22038/IJBMS.2017.9398.

65 Blázquez C, Carracedo A, Barrado L, et al. Cannabinoid receptors as novel targets for the treatment of melanoma. FASEB J. 2006;20(14):2633-5. doi:10.1096/fj.06-6638fje.

66 Armstrong JL, Hill DS, Mckee CS, et al. Exploiting cannabinoid-induced cytotoxic autophagy to drive melanoma cell death. J Invest Dermatol. 2015;135(6):1629-1637. doi: 10.1038/jid.2015.45.

67 Freimuth N, Ramer R, Hinz B. Antitumorigenic effects of cannabinoids beyond apoptosis. J Pharmacol Exp Ther. 2010;332(2):336-44. doi: 10.1124/jpet.109.157735.

68 Alshaarawy O, Anthony JC. Cannabis smoking and serum C-reactive protein: a quantile regressions approach based on NHANES 2005-2010. Drug Alcohol Depend. 2015;147:203-7. doi:10.1016/j.drugalcdep.2014.11.017.

69 Couch DG, Tasker C, Theophilidou E, et al. Cannabidiol and palmitoylethanolamide are anti-inflammatory in the acutely inflamed human colon. Clin Sci. 2017;131(21):2611-2626. doi: 10.1042/CS20171288.

70 Rodriguez-leyva D, Pierce GN. The cardiac and haemostatic effects of dietary hempseed. Nutr Metab (Lond). 2010;7:32. doi: 10.1186/1743-7075-7-32.

71 Vella RK, Jackson DJ, Fenning AS. Δ^9-Tetrahydrocannabinol prevents cardiovascular dysfunction in STZ-diabetic Wistar-Kyoto rats. Biomed Res Int. 2017;2017:7974149. doi: 10.1155/2017/7974149.

72 Chow L. It's official: 19 European countries say "no" to GMOs. EcoWatch. October 5, 2015. www.ecowatch.com/its-official-19-european-countries-say-no-to-gmos-1882106434.html. Accessed August 23, 2018.

73   Meyer N. Victory! Ireland doubles down on a GMO-free society, approves total ban on cultivation of GMO crops. March Against Monsanto. 12 July 2018. www.march-against-monsanto.com/victory-ireland-doubles-down-on-a-gmo-free-society-approves-total-ban-on-cultivation-of-gmo-crops/. Accessed August 23, 2018.

74   Miller J. Appeals court upholds California's Prop 65 glyphosate listing. Chemical Watch. April 25, 2018. https://chemicalwatch.com/66202/appeals-court-upholds-californias-prop-65-glyphosate-listing. Accessed August 23, 2018.

75   Meyer N. Del Bigtree, RFK lawsuit alleges complete failure to conduct necessary vaccine safety research over three decades-plus. July 16, 2018. www.march-against-monsanto.com/del-bigtree-rfk-lawsuit-alleges-hhs-completely-failed-to-conduct-vaccine-safety-research-over-30-plus-years/. Accessed August 23, 2018.

76   Kennedy RF, Baum K. "Monsanto's Roundup on trial: day 2 in court." Organic Consumers Association, 11 July 2018,. https://www.organicconsumers.org/blog/monsanto-roundup-cancer-trial

77   Meyer N. "BREAKING NEWS: The name Monsanto is officially history after 117 years of poisoning people around the globe." *March Against Monsanto*, 4 June 2018, www.march-against-monsanto.com/breaking-news-the-name-monsanto-is-officially-history-after-117-years-of-poisoning-people-around-the-globe/.

78   Cantani A. Benefits and concerns associated with biotechnology-derived foods: can additional research reduce children health risks?. Eur Rev Med Pharmacol Sci. 2009;13(1):41-50. https://www.ncbi.nlm.nih.gov/pubmed/19364084

79   De vendômois JS, Roullier F, Cellier D, et al. A comparison of the effects of three GM corn varieties on mammalian health. Int J Biol Sci. 2009;5(7):706-26. https://www.ncbi.nlm.nih.gov/pubmed/20011136

80   Smith J. Government Health Studies. Institute for Responsible Technology. https://responsibletechnology.org/government-studies/. Accessed August 23, 2018.

81   Samsel A, Seneff S. Glyphosate, pathways to modern diseases II: celiac sprue and gluten intolerance. Interdiscip Toxicol. 2013;6(4):159-84. doi: 10.2478/intox-2013-0026.

82   Samsel A, Seneff S. Glyphosate, pathways to modern diseases III: manganese, neurological diseases, and associated pathologies. Surg Neurol Int. 2015;6:45. 10.4103/2152-7806.153876.

83. Darien O. Pasteur versus Béchamp: the history of germ theory. Superlife: Hunting for Health. June 27, 2015. http://www.superlife.com/pasteur-bechamp-germ-theory/ Accessed August 23, 2018.

84   Costelloe C, Metcalfe C, Lovering A, et al. Effect of antibiotic prescribing in primary care on antimicrobial resistance in individual patients: systematic review and meta-analysis. BMJ. 2010;340:c2096. 10.1136/bmj.c2096.

85   Shehata AA, Schrödl W, Aldin AA, et al. The effect of glyphosate on potential pathogens and beneficial members of poultry microbiota in vitro. Curr Microbiol. 2013;66(4):350-8. doi: 10.1007/s00284-012-0277-2.

86   Bush Z. Redox molecule protection of tight junctions. Abstract of NIH Grant Application 1R43DK103422-01. Restore: New Earth Dynamics. No date. http://cdn.shopify.com/s/files/1/0354/2789/files/Abstract3.pdf?1413 Accessed August 23, 2018.

87   Rai M, Yadav A, Gade A. Silver nanoparticles as a new generation of antimicrobials. Biotechnol Adv. 2009;27(1):76-83. doi: 10.1016/j.biotechadv.2008.09.002.

ABOUT THE AUTHOR

Aaron Grosskopf

A aron is a Seattle native and at the start of grammar school, his father relocated the family to Napa, California. While growing up in the valley of food and wine, Aaron found his way into a kitchen at his first job with Kinyon Catering. Cooking would become desirable after high school and next, he found himself a student at Napa Valley Cooking school.

Upon graduation, Aaron worked at various restaurants in Napa, San Francisco, and New York City, under prestigious chefs in restaurants such as Domaine Chandon, Rubicon, Jardinere, 5th Floor, and the world famous Per Se. Early in his career, he ventured to Europe and staged at one star Michelin restaurant Pier Orsi, in Lyon, France.

Aaron then took another path and jumped into the private chef field in San Diego before moving back home to the Bay Area and San Francisco. During this time, a new desire came to the surface – natural health. Independently, he began this new path while still cooking, researching and studying alternative treatments. After using these methods in his own life, he began to reap the benefits and see others who were having the same successes. Then it came time to develop some street cred and put to use everything he learned over the years. He discovered IIN, the Institute for Integrative Nutrition. He took the Health Coach Training program and graduated as a Certified Health Coach.

As of this writing, Aaron is still cooking as a private chef with mobile gaming company Supercell, which has supported him in his pursuit to help others heal naturally. While working with clients as a health coach, the urge to write a book became strong. He wanted to share what he believes are tools anyone can use to turn their health around on their own, naturally. With that urge, *Don't Wait Until You're Sick* became a reality. He hopes you can use this information to your benefit and the benefit of others.

"Are your actions getting you closer to your goals?"

CPSIA information can be obtained
at www.ICGtesting.com
Printed in the USA
LVHW051045140122
708426LV00021B/2473

9 780578 403649